Reactions to Motherhood

The role of postnatal care

Jean A. Ball

MSc, Dip.N, RN, RM

Senior Teaching Fellow
Nuffield Institute for Health
University of Leeds

Books for Midwives Press
Books for Midwives Press is a joint publishing venture
between The Royal College of Midwives and
Haigh & Hochland Publications Ltd

Acknowledgements

This book would not have been written without the help of many people, to whom I wish to express my thanks. Firstly I would like to thank the 279 mothers who shared their experiences with me, and the midwives and obstetricians who allowed me to observe their work; the Department of Health and Social Security who funded the research, and Margorie and George Amans who provided me with hospitality and friendship.

My thanks also go to those who supervised the research: Dr Val Hillier in the Computation Department and Baroness McFarlance of Llandaff, Professor of Nursing, both in the Faculty of Medicine at Manchester University, and to Dr P Hawthorne of Nottingham University. Also to colleagues in the Marcé Society, especially Margaret Oates, John Cox and Channi Kumar.

Finally, my thanks and love must go to my personal support system, especially my husband Eric, whose unfailing support and patience has kept me going, and to my children Tim, Alison and Martin, who have become splendid people in spite of the mistakes their mother made!

Published by Books for Midwives Press, 174a Ashley Road, Hale, Cheshire, WA15 9SF, England

© 1994, Jean A. Ball

First edition

ISBN 1-898507-08-2

British Library Cataloguing in Publication Data
A catalogue record for this book is available from the British Library

Printed in Great Britain by Cromwell Press Ltd

Contents

Preface

The work upon which this book is based arose from a desire to learn more about the emotional needs of women as they take on the demanding role of motherhood, and to enable midwives to provide the kind of care which would best enhance the strengths and joys of women during this time.

My own training as a midwife had given me very little information about the psychological processes which underlie transition to motherhood: indeed most midwifery and obstetric textbooks lead one to assume that once a baby is safely born, the mother will instantly be able to cope with her new role. However, my experience as a midwife has shown me that women vary considerably in the adjustment to all that being a new mother brings.

The research which followed and which forms the basis of this book was designed to bridge those gaps; to learn more about the effects which psychological and social factors and the care given by midwives might have upon emotional needs of mothers during the first six weeks of their infants' lives; and to help midwives and other care-givers to make the emotional support of women an integral part of the care they give. The research traced the experiences of 279 women from the 36th week of pregnancy until six weeks after the birth of the baby, and included the perceptions which mothers and midwives had about each other and about the transition to motherhood.

Many different factors influence a woman's reactions to motherhood, and in order to understand the interaction of such factors and to evaluate the role played by postnatal care it was necessary to apply a strict discipline of statistical analysis to what is a funda-mentally subjective process. By this means I hoped to place the midwifery aspects of the study within the context of previous studies of the emotional reaction to mother-hood, and to avoid interpreting the results in line with my own feelings and cherished beliefs. The book contains, therefore, as much statistical evidence for its assertions as will satisfy the demands of a scientific approach to the subject, but not so much as to obscure the essence of the deeply personal experience of motherhood. I hope that those who are irritated by statistics will forgive their inclusion and perhaps appreciate their ability to illumine and add weight to argument and discussion, and that those who rely greatly upon them will appreciate that there are many things which cannot be measured.

Changes in knowledge since the first edition
The period when the research was undertaken and published concided with several significant studies of postnatal depression, which have considerably extended our un-derstanding of the factors associated with depression and emotional distress, and its potential impact upon the well-being of the baby. More specific measuring tools have been developed, and interventions which can reduce or alleviate postnatal depression evaluated.

A significant amount of this research has been undertaken in the United Kingdom, and thus provides a framework within which the midwifery research aspects can be com-pared and discussed. Happily, there are sufficient parallels between the different stud-ies to make this possible. This second edition, therefore, will review much of this research and discuss the results in the light of it.

Another important development has been the establishment of the Marcé Society*, which has been instrumental in disseminating information and stimulating multidisciplinary interest in the emotional and mental health of childbearing women; and the establish-ment of voluntary organizations such as the Association for Postnatal Illness.

However, there is still very little research into the effects which midwifery care may have upon the emotional needs of women. This is surprising when one considers that midwives support mothers through the childbearing process in all societies and have done so since the beginning of recorded history! If the misery of emotional distress and depression which affects so many women after the birth of a baby is to be reduced, then we must continue to expand our understanding of the processes and skills which will provide personal, sensitive and life-enhancing care to mothers, their babies and part-ners, and to ensure that the way in which the maternity services are organized provides an enriching and equitable service to all.

CHAPTER 1

Birth and Change

The birth of a baby is an eagerly awaited event. It is also the beginning of major change in the life of its parents. Whilst both parents must now undertake new roles and responsibilities, the mother is the one most profoundly affected. Many demands will be made upon her during the period immediately following the birth. During the time of recovery from the physical stress of pregnancy and labour she will experience conflicting emotions of joy and anxiety as she becomes aware of the utter dependence of her infant upon her, and the responsibility which is now hers. She must learn and master new skills in feeding and caring for her baby, and both she and her partner must come to terms with the social restrictions which caring for a new baby requires. Nor are these transient changes, for this child, and any other children which they may have, will need its parents' care and commitment for many years if his or her full potential is to be realized.

The enormous demands of parenthood

As childbirth is such a common experience, it is perhaps easy to overlook the tremendous and unique changes which it brings. One of these is the irrevocable nature of the physical processes of pregnancy, labour and birth. Birth, like death, cannot be avoided. Successful pregnancy leads on to the inevitability of labour, which cannot be stopped or started at will, but which takes over the mother completely. There is no going back.

The process of pregnancy and parenthood can be said to involve a series of losses; loss of control over one's physical state, loss of control over lifestyle and the loss of sleep which caring for a small baby brings. Against this must be set the gains; the joy and delight which a new child brings, the fulfilment of the desire to become a family, the change in status within the family, as "children" become parents, and "parents" become grandparents. Such tremendous changes require a period of adjustment and adaptation, and the significance of these events for the family and the wider society, are marked in most cultures by a variety of rituals and rites of passage (Cox, 1988; Kitzinger, 1989).

The birth of a baby is, therefore, not only the beginning of the infant's life; it is also a major life-change, bringing about a new pattern of life for the whole family. The pattern which emerges will be influenced by the thoughts, beliefs, personalities and attitude of the people involved, and by the values of the society in which they live.

Life-change and stress

Any major life-change provokes some degree of stress. Holmes and Rahe (1967) devised a rating scale which lists 43 major life-events in order of the degree of stress with which they are associated. Whilst the death of a spouse is listed as the most stressful life-event, pregnancy and the acquisition of a new family member are both included within the first 20. For some couples, a number of other major life-events may be occurring at the same time as pregnancy and the birth of a baby. These may include marriage, changes in financial status, the woman giving up her work, the acquisition of a mortgage, and a change of home. It is small wonder that Brown (1979) described childbirth and the puerperium as uniquely stressful among normal expected life experiences. It must be remembered however, that the list produced by Holmes and Rahe (1967) was related to the general public and therefore did not include the positive and fulfilling life-changes of motherhood. A number of studies of postnatal depression have adapted the Holmes and Rahe scale and this will be discussed more fully later. However, it would be true to say that we do not yet understand the degree to which other "positive" life-changes may counterbalance stressful life-events.

Adaptation to change

Many women will adapt to motherhood and its demands with a minimum of stress because of their own psychological strengths and the quality of the support they receive from their family and friends. Others will experience severe stress during the transition to motherhood. Some of these will arise from the woman's own psychological needs; others will be caused by external factors such as financial difficulties, a demanding older child, or marital tension. The experience of hospitalization, too, is stressful to most people, as it causes them to relinquish control over their patterns of daily living. During this time the way in which care is given by professional care-givers should be sensitive and related to individual needs. It should be designed to enhance the mother's particular strengths and confidence, and at the very least should avoid the addition of extra stress by insensitive attitudes or approaches to care. If care-givers are to fulfil this function, they will need to understand something of the psychological processes involved in adjusting to change and coping with stress. The experience of parenting is a mixed blessing and will provoke a number of conflicting reactions and feelings.

> Being a mother is harder work than I had imagined it to be. I now realize that a baby definitely is not a doll to be paraded around in fancy frills!
>
> At times he is a real handful, and when my husband goes to work after a rough night I feel very depressed and unable to cope. I find that when he has been upset all day I am watching the clock and waiting for my husband to come home, and feel relieved when he does.
>
> But when the baby is awake and looking at me and learning to use his arms and legs, or asleep in my arms, I get a feeling of utter peace and contentment and realize he is worth it after all.
>
> (Glenis, aged 23, first-time mother)

Every individual has a continuing need for physical safety, love and security, esteem and achievement (Maslow, 1970). The satisfaction of these needs produces a state of emotional security which can be described as an internal feeling-state of confidence and emotional well-being. The experiences of living involve adapting to numerous changes and many different situations. As a result we develop attitudes and patterns of behaviour which enable us to maintain our state of emotional well-being, and through the development of these patterns we are able to achieve desired objectives, and to develop the maturity to accept disappointment and failure.

When major life-changes occur, or when the normal mechanisms for dealing with change and challenge are not effective, some degree of stress will be experienced until the disturbing situation has been dealt with and overcome. The way in which an individual deals with such a situation has been called the 'coping process' (Lazarus, 1969). This process is recognized as having a consistent pattern.

Demands, needs and reactions

Lazarus describes the two main forms of demand which are made on the individual and affect their response to change of stress.

1.   The individual's internal needs, which are derived from his or her personality, previous experiences and desire for approval and achievement.
2.   External demands and expectations of behaviour which arise from peer values, the culture and society to which a person belongs.

The way these different demands interact with each other to form the basis of the coping response. Lazarus also emphazises that the type of coping behaviour which is adopted by the individual must be understood in terms of a transaction between the individual concerned, the stress being experienced, and the environment in which coping is taking place.

This relationship between the internal and external demands made on an individual during adjustment to change is taken a stage further by Caplan (1964), who describes three groups of needs which must be met if emotional equilibrium is to be maintained. These are the physical needs of safety, food and shelter, the need for personal interaction with others in the family or peer group, and the need to react within the constraints set by the social and cultural mores of the society in which the individual lives.

Emotions

In all these complex interactions of internal needs and external pressures, strong emotions will be experienced. Emotions are powerful forces which affect perception, understanding, behaviour and attitudes. The effect of emotion will be seen during the period of adjustment to stress and as an end product of the coping process. Nor should it be thought that 'emotions' mean only the weepiness and distress which is sometimes associated with women; emotions also include joy and love, and can be life-enriching and positive. The event of marriage is listed seventh in Holmes and Rahe's list of stressful life-events, and the amount of adjustment required by both partners in a marriage is well recognized. Nevertheless, marriage is usually accompanied by emotions of joy and happiness. Similarly a mother's delight in her child can enable her to overcome considerable physical discomfort and psychological stress. This is an under-researched aspect of factors associated with adjustment to motherhood. We simply do not know the extent to which the generally observed delight of mothers in their babies affects their reaction to the "increasingly complex interaction between sociocultural, psychological and biological changes surrounding childbirth" (Cox, 1988). If the mother's delight in her child does indeed act as a protecting factor, then studies which disregard its potential or compare the incidence of depression in postnatal women with that of non-puerperal women without acknowledging its influence may be overlooking a vital factor (O'Hara *et al*, 1984).

Support systems and care-givers

Another important component in the transactional process of adjusting to change and stress is that of the availability and quality of support. Caplan (1964) considers that people experiencing major upheaval in their lives are more susceptible to the influence of others than they are at times of normal functioning, and that the quality of the support given by others may have the effect of 'loading the dice' in favour of a good or poor outcome. He argues, therefore, that all of the caring professions "need to develop their knowledge and technical insight in order to practice more surely the kind of work which will help clients emotionally and mentally, as well as achieving the basic goals of the profession".

Midwives and companions

Women have always sought the help of their female companions during the time of childbirth and mothering, and such records as exist reflect the effect that the culture to which both mother and midwife belonged had upon their relationship with each other. Thus, we read in Genisis 35: v.16-20 that the midwife caring for Rachel during her last and fatal labour, sought to strengthen and encourage her dying patient with the news that she had borne Jacob yet another son, that great status symbol of the Jewish tribe. In more recent years, male-dominated Victorian society, scandalized at the use of chloroform in relieving labour pains because it 'robbed God of the deep and earnest cries of women in the pains of childbirth', had to change its attitudes overnight when Queen Victoria used chloroform for the birth of her eighth child in 1852! Such luxuries were only for the wealthy and influential, however. A remarkable collection of letters from working women which was first published in 1915 gives striking examples of the miseries of childbirth and motherhood endured in poverty and made worse by the 'modesty' which prevented 'respectable' women from seeking help in the prevention of unwanted pregnancies (Llewellyn Davies, 1979). These letters were collected as part of a campaign to provide a free midwifery service which would give care to mothers either in their own homes or in local maternity homes. Since that time the maternity services for women in the United Kingdom have grown and developed beyond all expectations. In that time there has been great change in both the style and methods of delivering those services. De Vries (1989) suggests that maternity care has moved from being passive, to active, and then to controlled. The passive phase of care was dominated by the midwife, and gave way to the increasingly active and doctor led "scientific" approach with the almost universal switch from home to hospital. He contends that as birth became less dangerous and yielded better results, it was possible to move into the controlled stage, characterized by increased concern for the experiential elements of birth.

Midwives and mothers continue to play their complementary roles, even though birth now takes place within the setting of a maternity hospital. Midwives take full responsibility for the labour and delivery of the majority of mothers in the United Kingdom: they run the labour suites, the postnatal wards and the special care baby units; they visit mothers on a daily basis after discharge from hospital for at least ten days after the birth and often for a longer period. It would seem reasonable to suppose, therefore, that the care given to mothers by midwives during this time has an important part to play in enabling women to adjust successfully to the demands which motherhood makes upon them and their families. It is surprising that so little attention has been given to the way in which postnatal care is organized and to the relationships between mothers and midwives during the crucial first days and weeks following the birth of a baby.

This book is based upon research designed to increase knowledge of the effects which midwives working within the National Health Service may or may not have upon the ability of mothers to adjust to the demands of the postnatal period. The design of the research was based upon the premise that women react to childbirth and motherhood in the same way that people react to any major life-change, and therefore explored the psychological concepts underlying the processes of coping and adjustment in order to identify factors which were likely to affect reactions to motherhood. Previous studies exploring factors related to postnatal depression, and those concerned with factors affecting the development of maternal-child relationships were also considered, as it is only when these factors are more fully understood that the role played by the midwife be evaluated.

CHAPTER 2

Factors Involved in the Coping Process

Stress and coping

The word "stress" is used widely. In colloquial terms it is used to convey some degree of harassment, heavy workload or the problems of meeting many and varied demands. The term stress has a dual meaning, it may describe the provoking situation or problem as well as the state of tension which is felt until the problem has receded or is overcome.

Arnold (1960) defined stress as any condition which disturbs normal functioning. Normal functioning, of course, varies considerably from person to person according to the factors and events which have contributed to each individual's unique situation. These factors include personality, previous experiences and the particular situation in which stress is being experienced.

It is vital that care-givers understand that a person's reactions to stress are governed by a multiplicity of internal and external factors, and that although emotions displayed appear to have been provoked by a particular event, they really reflect the results of a complex process, many of the features of which are outside the control of either the individual concerned or the care-giver.

If we take Arnold's definition, then it could be said that any major change affecting a person will "disturb normal functioning" to a lesser or greater degree. If the change is prolonged or permanent, then it will give rise to a period of adjustment during which the person adapts to the new environment or situation. If the change has been sought after, or is seen as beneficial b y the subject, then the process of adjustment will be comparatively easy. However, there may be factors in the situation which bring unexpected stress.

The way in which a person responds to change or stress has been described as the "coping process" (Lazarus, 1966). Lazarus distinguishes between the terms 'coping' and 'adjustment'; he defines coping as coming to terms with a situation, but adjustment as exerting mastery over it. Success in achieving some degree of coping will eventually lead to full adjustment.

Factors which influence the coping process

Lazarus described a number of factors which influence the coping process and which influence its outcome in terms of coping or mastery, and these are listed below.

- Antecedent factors which predispose the way individuals respond to change. These include personality, previous learning experience, the degree of success or failure in coping in the past, beliefs or expectations of one's ability to adjust to the change and achieve the desired outcome.
- The degree of stress being experienced, either in the provoking situation or arising from the tension experienced in trying to deal with it.
- The quality of the support upon which the individual is able to draw.

During this process of coping and readjustment, new skills are learned, and existing attitudes or beliefs may be reinforced or weakened. Patterns of behaviours which have been successful in the past will be adopted, and if successful they will be continued. However, if they do not prove successful, then the person must find some other way of handling the situation, and this can cause further anxiety and tension until the situation is under control.

Factors affecting the coping process

Antecedent factors: personality and previous experiences

The main antecedent factors involved in the coping process are personality and previous learning experiences. Freud (1940) considered that the major facets of personality are fixed before the age of five years and that little change is possible after that age. Other psychologists argue that personality continues to develop from birth onwards, going through a number of identifiable stages which are influenced by the learning process (Erikson, 1963). Some of those stages are particularly pertinent to the situation of parenthood. Erikson described the "early adult" stage as culminating in the ability to form intimate and lasting relationships and to make long-term commitments.

The effect of personality on adjustment to motherhood has been considered by a number of researchers and will be discussed in greater detail later. Perhaps the most notable study was that by Pitt (1968), on a sample of 305 mothers. He found that ten per cent of them were depressed six weeks post-partum. Pitt had assessed the personality of the mothers during the last trimester of pregnancy and found that those who had high trait anxiety formed a significant proportion of those later found to be depressed. Similar effects have been found in the reactions of patients admitted for non-urgent reasons to medical wards. Wilson-Barnett (1979) found that patients with a high trait anxiety took much longer to adjust to the hospital environment than did those with normal or low levels of anxiety.

Previous experiences

Previous experiences also influence the coping process. They affect the perception of the situation, the individual's belief in his or her ability to cope, and the motivation needed to adapt to and master the new circumstances.

People who have been "successful" in the past are likely to tackle the situation of change with confidence. However, those whose experience has not been so fortunate may feel afraid, or experience some degree of helplessness when faced with a difficult situation.

A very interesting set of studies by Seligman (1975) demonstrated that where subjects were unable to avoid or deal successfully with a stressful situation they tended to slip into apathy and gave up any further attempts to avoid the stress. For them, 'taking the punishment' was preferable to further failure at overcoming the painful situation. When the same subjects were later put into a situation in which avoidance and escape were possible, they made no attempt to do either, but accepted the situation and again 'took the punishment'. The prospect of failing yet again was apparently more painful than the stress to which they were subjected, and the key factor appeared to be their belief that they were unable to control the situation in which they were placed. This was defined as "learned helplessness", and this degree of apathy and inaction can be seen as a form of coping behaviour but not one which is to be desired.

Anxiety

Anxiety may be seen at any stage of the coping process, either as an antecedent factor, as a reaction, or as a continuing feature of individual coping behaviour.

There are two main forms of anxiety - trait anxiety and state anxiety - and it is important to realize that both may be operating in a given situation. Trait anxiety is a stable personality trait, whereas state anxiety is a transitory fluctuating response to the perception of danger or threat (Cattell and Scheier, 1961). Most people are familiar with some of the physical manifestations of state anxiety such as a dry mouth, sweating palms and 'butterflies in the tummy'.

Anxiety affects both perception and understanding. Anxious people are less able to take in information and instruction and tend to blame themselves for their lack of understanding. Midwives may well remember their own reactions of anxiety and distress when becoming a student midwife after working as either a staff nurse or ward sister in general nursing. Many midwives recall the unhappiness and loss of self-esteem which resulted when their previous experience and level of competence were regarded as irrelevant in this new situation. During this period of anxiety they found that the attitude of certain qualified midwives reinforced their feelings of incompetence and further reduced their ability to learn the new skills expected of them. Coping behaviour in this situation usually took the form of avoiding such qualified staff, quickly 'learning the ropes' in order to avoid further stress, and depending very greatly on the support of other students on the same course. The situation which is related by most midwives amply illustrates the primary and secondary reactions to stress described by psychologists and enables us to appreciate both the effects which stress has upon normal functioning, and the way our support systems enable us to overcome stress. Eventually, of course, most student midwives master the new skills expected of them, enabling them in retrospect to laugh at the painful experience. It is notable, however, that very few ever forget it.

External factors which may affect the process

As Lazarus (1966) has noted, the outcome of the coping process arises from a transaction between the individual, and the circumstances which give rise to the stress. The work of Holmes and Rahe (1967) have shown the way in which a major life-change or a series of smaller life changes in combination, can affect mental and physical well-being. Therefore a person's previous ability to cope successfully may be undermined by a major stressful event or by some comparatively minor event which acts as "the straw that broke the camel's back". It will be vital therefore to reduce or prevent any unnecessary additional stress and protecting the affected person from such difficulties is particularly the function of the support system upon which he or she can rely.

The significance of support systems

> A man does not face crisis alone but is helped or hindered by the people around him, by his family, his friends, neighbourhood, community and nation. (Caplan, 1964)

Lazarus (1969) also places great emphasis on the need to understand the coping process in the context of the individual's environment. This sociocultural environment affects the process of coping through its effects upon personality, perception and cognition, and the constraints which its values place upon a person's behaviour. For example, the experience of bereavement is common to all societies, but the expression of grief ranges from the stiff upper lip of the British to the wailing distress of Eastern cultures. It is probable that cultures which allow grief to be expressed and shared, help the bereaved person to come to terms with the situation better than those which treat death as an unmentionable subject and thus leave the bereaved person isolated.

The degree to which the sociocultural environment affects adjustment to motherhood has been explored by some researchers. In her study of present day birth rituals in both developing and Western societies, Kitzinger (1978, 1989) concluded that all maternal behaviour is culturally determined. Oakley (1980) considered that its influence had been seriously neglected by many researchers in this field. Part of the reason for this lack, is the difficulty in gaining sufficient funding for the detailed and research-intensive work over large samples which are required to obtain robust information (Reid and Garcia, 1989).

Within the broad aspects of the sociocultural climate is embedded the particular support system surrounding an individual, and the degree to which that support provides the right counterbalance to the antecedent and stress factors affecting the coping patterns.

The significance of the support system

The supportive environment, therefore, can be seen to have some role to play in influencing a person's adjustment to change and stress. In fact, if the antecedent factors which predispose the coping reaction are permanent or semi-permanent features of an individual's make-up, then the only variable factor in the coping process is that of the environment in which change is being faced. This support comes in the forms of peers, family, professional and lay helpers, the services provided by society as a whole. It is therefore one factor in the coping process which may be most readily improved in order to enable the individual to achieve a healthy outcome. This has been highlighted in various studies into the factors affecting maternal-child relationships in the early postnatal period. Klaus and Kennell (1970, 1976, 1982) demonstrated that the attitudes and practices of hospital staff could be changed in order to provide an environment which enhanced rather than hindered the attachment process between mother and baby. Later research (Klaus et al, 1986) has demonstrated that continuous social support can also affect the physical outcome of labour for both mother and baby.

What is support?

The term 'support' is freely used in nursing and medical reports, but its meaning in relation to the individual patient is often not defined. Caplan and Killilea (1976) define support as 'an enduring pattern of continuous or intermittent ties that play a significant part in maintaining the psychological and physical integrity of the individual over time'. Whilst the support provided for an individual by his or her family is of paramount importance, that offered by peer, friend, professional helpers and social institutions may also make a considerable difference to emotional well-being and coping ability. Weiss (1976) defines effective support as that given by a person, either professional or lay, who is accepted as an ally by the distressed person. The helper's acceptance will depend upon the ability to convince the distressed person that his or her training and experience, understanding and commitment are available for as long as they are needed. This, in turn, will depend on a two-way exchange of information and mutual trust, and the development of a relationship between the helper and the person needing help. The role of the helper is to listen as well as to instruct, and to give help which is relevant to the needs of the individual rather than in compliance with a preconceived model of how that person should react.

When considering the role of support systems in the adjustment of women to childbirth and motherhood, it is interesting to note that many studies in this area have either concentrated upon factors in the mother which are related to postnatal depression without considering her environment, or have criticised the hospital environment without considering the factors in the mother which were related to postnatal depression or would have affected her reaction to hospitalization.

The growth among mothers of self-help groups such as the National Childbirth Trust and the La Leche League may be indications of the failure of family or professional helpers to provide appropriate support. They illustrate that relationship between the helper and the individual being helped that is described by Weiss (1976). They also exert an influence upon the mother's behaviour by their values and the emphasis placed upon certain aspects of motherhood such as breastfeeding. This may lead to their membership mainly consisting of women with similar attitudes and values, but their success nevertheless amply illustrates the value of an acceptable and appropriate support system.

Effects upon outcomes

An understanding of the role which a support system may have in influencing the outcome of the coping process leads to a realization that no set pattern or routine provision can meet the needs of all individuals. Whilst the initial reaction to stress will be profoundly affected for good or ill by the fixed antecedent factors of personality, previous experiences and expectations, the professional helper can influence the situation by the appropriateness of the help provided (Currell, 1990) and the sensitivity with which it is given (Flint, 1986). Such help should, therefore, be flexible in its approach and degree.

The support system surrounding women during pregnancy, labour and childbirth consists of family and peers, and the maternity services provided by the society in which the woman lives. In the United Kingdom this service is given via the National Health Service and spans care given by general practitioners, midwives and health visitors in the primary care team, and obstetricians, paediatricians, midwives, anaesthetists and physiotherapists in the hospital services.

The developments in medicine and technology designed to reduce perinatal and maternal mortality have mainly taken place during the last 30 years, and have thereby changed social and family patterns of support for childbirth which had been in existence for many centuries. In the United Kingdom, 99 per cent of all births now take place in hospitals or GP maternity units. Among other things this means that for many women their first experience of hospitalization coincides with the experience of childbirth and motherhood. There is a danger that those of us who spend our working lives in the hospital environment may not appreciate the stress which admission to hospital and the loss of control over patterns of daily living can cause to patients.

The manner in which maternity care is provided has been the focus of discussion in recent years, and the report of the Social Services Committee on Perinatal and Maternal Mortality (House of Commons 1980) pointed out that the emotional support given to mothers was of major importance. It went on to say that any mother who produced a healthy baby but looked back on the experience as one she would not want to repeat should be regarded as evidence of failure of the service!

Within this total service to women, midwives play a major role. Not only are they the professional group whose work is exclusively concerned with child-bearing women, they are the principal providers of care during labour, delivery and the postnatal period. Reactions to motherhood may begin in pregnancy, but they become apparent after the birth. The support given by midwives to mothers may have a significant contribution to make, and it is for this reason that the research described in later chapters sought to evaluate the effects of postnatal care provided by midwives upon maternal emotional well-being during the puerperium.

Understanding coping behaviour

The way people react to any stressful change or situation will depend upon their internal needs, which may include some of the antenatal factors noted earlier, and will initially follow their usual patterns of dealing with challenges. Lazarus (1966) describes four main forms of coping behaviour, all of which are designed to enable the person concerned to cope with a stressful situation which is not yet overcome. These are listed below.

- Anticipatory action
- Attack
- Avoidance
- Apathy and inaction

The first two forms of behaviour; anticipatory action and attack, are designed to gain some degree of control over situation. Avoidance implies some degree of denial or prudence, but the last is indicative of being unable to deal successfully with the stress being experienced.

Anticipatory action

Anticipatory action implies some degree of planning and preparing for an expected event, finding out as much as possible in advance and taking steps to reduce stress which arises from the unknown. This can be seen in the way people prepare for exams or interviews. It would be reasonable to consider that pregnancy is a time when anticipatory action in preparing for the baby, and the experience of feeling the baby move, begins the adjustment process. Attendance at parentcraft classes, visiting the delivery suite, drawing up birth plans and discussing expectations and fears about the labour all play a part in this coping strategy. As this type of preparation is or should be available to all women it highlights the importance of antenatal information and the building of trusting relationships between the consumer and the care-providers. It is vital therefore that birth plans and the mother's wishes are not ignored or rejected unless some major problem intervenes.

Attack

Attack is a powerful coping strategy designed to gain control over a situation, by exerting powerful influences, to concentrate one's resources, to impose will. People with dominant or dominating personalities, and those who are used to exerting authority over others may respond in this way. The means of expressing this form of coping will be constrained by social and cultural values.

Mothers (and midwives?) who insist on a rigid routine of baby care or housework may be using attack as the means of coping with a situation which might otherwise be overwhelming. Likewise, the existence and activities of certain pressure groups that want to change the present patterns of maternity care may arise from the stresses produced in their members during pregnancy and childbirth. While most such groups make informed and constructive criticisms of the professionals concerned, attack as a form of coping may be seen in the consistently destructive criticism expressed by a few individuals.

Avoidance

Avoidance as a coping behaviour can be regarded as prudent, by avoiding situations which the individual knows will be difficult to handle, or as opting out or denial of a stressful situation. Students may find plausible excuses for dropping a difficult course of study; children may run away from an unhappy home. The large number of people who 'disappear' every year, leaving behind their homes, families and livelihood also illustrates avoidance behaviour. Suicide can be seen as avoidance behaviour in its most extreme form, and agoraphobia as avoidance of the fear-provoking world outside the safe home environment.

The 'learned helplessness' found by Seligman (1975) showed that vulnerable animals and human beings preferred to accept a painful situation rather than experience the pain of failure once again. They avoided making the effort to get out of the painful situation because the recurrence of failure would form a greater threat to their self-esteem. The reluctance of some women to attend antenatal clinics in hospital may not be a rejection of the expertise offered at such clinics, but avoidance of the stress incurred by the difficulties of making a long journey to the hospital, coping with older children during the visit, or the experience of being deprived of personal clothing and identity as they pass along the antenatal clinic conveyor belt. All of these factors may combine to make non-attendance an appropriate form of coping.

Apathy and inaction

Continuing patterns of being unable to overcome a stressful situation can lead to persistent apathy and inaction. Coping with stress may have physiological as well as psychological effects. Stress has been recognized as a contributory factor in the formation of stomach ulcers and in heart disease.

Lazarus defines inaction as, "the complete absence of any impulse to deal with a situation". Hilgard, Atkinson and Atkinson (1979) give the example of concentration camp victims, for whom apathy and inaction had become such a persistent behavioural pattern that they were totally unable to respond to their liberation by allied troops at the end of the war. Increased understanding of the causes of apathy and inaction may help midwives to understand why some mothers with multiple social problems do not seek help until pregnancy is well advanced or until labour itself begins, and to devise strategies for care which can help to overcome these difficulties (Evans, 1988).

Depression

Apathy and inaction can be seen as symptoms of depression (Lazarus, 1966). Dalton (1980) describes depression as a disease of loss, characterized by gloom, despondency and despair. This kind of depression is known as reactive depression. In their influential study of the social causes of depression in women, Brown and Harris (1978) found that working class women were more likely to suffer depression because of their lack of control over their lives. Of these women, those with two or more small children to care for, and who lacked the comfort of a "warm, confiding relationship" with their husband or a male partner, were the most vulnerable. Victims of depression experience the loss of happiness, pleasure, interest and enthusiasm, as well as the ability to think clearly, to concentrate or to remember. Other losses may include appetite, sleep, weight control and bowel movement.

Emotional reactions to the demands of motherhood

When the various factors involved in coping with major upheavals in life are considered it is not perhaps surprising that some women suffer postnatal depression. Indeed, one might wonder why all women do not suffer from it. Postnatal depression is one end of a whole spectrum of emotional reactions to motherhood. At the other end is the happy, fulfilled and well-adjusted mother who delights in her new status and role. In-between are the majority of women who calmly adjust to motherhood without experiencing the euphoria of one extreme or the depression of the other.

CHAPTER 3

Reactions to Motherhood

What is motherhood?

Perhaps the first stage in seeking to understand reactions to motherhood is to define what we mean by this term. It might be said that it is almost impossible to define fully what motherhood means to a woman. In terms of an event or process it might be defined as a physiological and psychological process which leads to and underpins the experience of giving birth and nurturing a child, and which provokes strong emotions. Page (1988) reflects on the mixture of feelings, "the ambivalence, the wretchedness of morning sickness, the joy, the anxiety, the disappointment and the family disruptions of pregnancy". She goes on to say that the event is physical, but also sexual and spiritual, "full of a range of emotions; happiness and joy, fear, anxiety, anger and frustration, grief and poignancy ... joy and ecstasy and infinite tenderness". In view of the overwhelming and all embracing nature of this experience, it seems impertinent to suggest that there might be a "normal" period of time within which a woman is able to adjust to her new role, and yet, there seems to be a tacit assumption that such a time exists. But what period of time is "right" and what pattern of care will best enable a woman to gain mastery over all the demands of motherhood?

In 1902 in the United Kingdom, the legislation surrounding midwifery practice set ten days as the required time of "lying-in" after the birth, during which time the mother was expected to rest and to receive attention from a midwife. It seems that women valued this time highly (Llewellyn Davies, 1979; Houldsworth, 1988). Since that time developments in maternity care and the routines of hospital practice have created other time targets, e.g. discharge from hospital around 48 hours after the birth for the majority of women, albeit with further care from the community midwife. Many women now resume household duties by the end of the first week after the birth and very few have the benefit of female relatives living nearby. Other societies, however, do not demand so much from their mothers. Cox (1988) notes that in China, mothers are given a month off all household duties after giving birth and are "treated as a queen" before taking on the full care of the baby or the household. He wonders whether studies in China might show reduced levels of postnatal depression because of this.

In fact, we have no real basis for assuming that there is any period which could be considered to be the "proper" time within which a woman s*hould* be able to adjust to the demands of motherhood, but social, family and health service patterns do seem to assume that most women should be coping with motherhood within a few weeks of childbirth. Many studies of postnatal depression have taken six weeks post-delivery as the time for assessing emotional outcome. In most cases this has been chosen for convenience because it coincides with the time of the postnatal physical check-up, and on the face of it, it does seem to be a reasonable time in which most women will indeed find themselves able to cope successfully. However, there is no evidence that this time is the "normal" time for adjustment, some mothers will be coping much earlier, others will need longer before they feel in control of their situation.

Understanding reactions to motherhood

The research was designed to examine whether different patterns of postnatal care provided by midwives had any effect upon the way women reacted to the major life-event of becoming a mother. Although evidence from studies of postnatal depression formed an important part of the research planning, the study did not focus only on those women who had negative outcomes in terms of depression but considered all the different ranges of emotional well-being and sought to highlight any factors which proved to be significant in distinguishing between women who were happy and coping well, those who were content, coping but not euphoric about motherhood and those who were unhappy, distressed or depressed.

It was vital, therefore, to include within the study, those factors which had been found to be significant in studies of postnatal depression. In 1980, when the research was planned, several notable studies had been published (Pitt, 1968; Cox, 1978; Kumar and Robson, 1978) but others which have made important contributions to our understanding (Paykel, 1980; Cox et al, 1987; Kumar and Robson, 1984), were still in process. At that time, almost all the research on emotional outcomes of childbirth lay in the realm of studies of postnatal depression, and to a lesser degree in studies of factors influencing maternal-infant relationships in the immediate post-birth period (Klaus and Kennel, 1976). Very few studies had considered the impact of support systems.

Emotional/psychological reactions to motherhood

Three main types of emotional or mental disturbance following childbirth are recognized; the postnatal blues, postnatal depression and puerperal psychosis. These have been explained fully elsewhere (Cox, 1986; Brockington and Cox-Roper, 1988; O'Hara and Zekoski, 1988; Affonso, 1984; Arizmendi and Affonso, 1984; Romito, 1989). The blues are regarded as a transitory mood disturbance which affects 70-80 per cent of all mothers within a day or two of delivery, postnatal depression affects between 10-20 per cent of all mothers and is primarily regarded as reactive depression (see Table 3.1). Puerperal psychosis is comparatively and mercifully rare affecting about one per cent of all mothers.

Studies of postnatal depression

Although some researchers have recently questioned whether postnatal depression is any different from that which affects women at other times in their lives O'Hara et al, 1990; Cox et al, 1993), it is generally regarded as unique, because it follows childbirth, and it is thought to have "atypical" signs and symptoms (Pitt, 1968; Dalton, 1980). This perception has been strengthened by the controlled study by Cox et al (1993) which compared depression in parturient and non-parturient women, and found a greatly increased onset of depression occurring within one month of delivery in the parturient women. Cox concludes that "this was a direct consequence of the physical and psychological stresses of childbirth".

Table 3.1: Sample size and incidence of postnatal depression/distress in five studies

Author/date	Sample size	Time of assessment (post-partum)	Depressed (%)
Pitt, 1968, UK	305	6-8 weeks	10.8 +10 'distressed'
Paykel *et al*, 1980, UK	120	5-8 weeks	20
Cox *et al*, 1982, UK	105	4 months	13
Cox, 1983, Uganda and UK	183	3 months	10
Kumar and Robson, 1984, UK	119	3 months 12 months	14 23% of above were still depressed

Another unique aspect of postnatal depression is the impact this illness has upon the family, and if severe or extended, there is growing evidence that it has a negative effect upon the interpersonal and emotional development of the infant (Murray, 1988) and on the cognitive development of the older child (Cogill *et al*, 1986). When one considers that most studies show an incidence of 10-20 per cent of mothers suffering depression, then at 600,000 births per annum in the United Kingdom, one can expect between 60,000 and 120,000 families to be adversely affected.

In his classic study, Pitt (1968) described postnatal depression as "atypical" and accompanied by tearfulness, despondency, feelings of inadequacy and inability to cope, together with feelings of anxiety about the baby and guilt linked to self-reproach at not caring for or loving the baby properly. He notes that in almost every case, the mothers were in fact, providing very good care for their babies, who were all thriving. Dalton (1980) described postnatal depression as having features which distinguish it from other types of depression. Most depressed people may get off to sleep successfully but then wake in the early hours and are unable to get back to sleep again. Women with postnatal depression, however, have a great need of sleep and cannot get enough of it. They tend to sleep heavily, waking to attend to the baby and can then sleep on throughout the night and during the day if the opportunity occurs. Most depressed people dread the mornings, but depressed mothers are at their best in the morning and feel progressively worse as the day goes on.

Early studies of emotional outcomes of childbirth

It is intriguing to note that certain early studies of "maladjustment" to motherhood sought to explain women's reactions in terms of their "femininity". In a description of maternal emotions, Newton (1955) explored the feelings of women towards menstruation, pregnancy and childbirth, breastfeeding, caring for an infant and "other aspects of their femininity" with the clear inference that "feminine" women would feel positive about these experiences Chertok (1969) and Nilsson (1972) both produced scales of "femininity" from which they attempted to show that postnatal depression was related to a woman's rejection of her feminine role in childbirth. One wonders that the reaction would be if it was suggested that men who suffered depression following trauma were somehow lacking in their masculinity! The majority of studies, however, began to identify stress factors in relation to postnatal depression and many of these can be seen in Table 3.2.

Table 3.2: Factors associated with postnatal depression/distress from several studies

Factor	Found to be significant	Not found to be sigificant
Obstetric problems	Oakley, 1980 (small sample, linked to dissatisfaction with birth management	Pitt, 1968; Paykel *et al*, 1980; Kumar and Robson, 1984 Stein *et al*, 1989
Parity	Pitt, 1968 (more in primiparae)	Paykel, 1980; Cox, 1983
Poor relationship/ separation from own mother	Frommer and O'Shea, 1973; Kumar and Robson, 1984	Paykel, 1980
Unplanned pregnancy		Paykel, 1980
Marital conflict	Paykel, 1980; Oakley, 1980; Kumar and Robson, 1984; Watson, 1984; O'Hara *et al*, 1983	
Lack of confidante	Stein *et al*, 1989	
Life-events in year preceding pregnancy	Paykel, 1980; Watson, 1984; Cooper *et al*, 1988	
Social class		Paykel, 1980; Watson, 1984
Social problems	Stein *et al*, 1989	

Tod (1964) studied 700 women of whom he judged three per cent to be depressed to a degree which required psychiatric intervention. All the depressed women had shown marked anxiety during the pregnancy, came from poor family and social backgrounds and had some degree of abnormal obstetric history, This percentage of three per cent of a large sample is very low when compared with other studies which show a percentage of 10-20 per cent depressed mothers, but this may have been due to Tod's stringent definition of depression. Tod's results were very similar to those of Brown and Harris, whose study was of depression in women in general. In their major study of the social causes of depression in women they found that those most vulnerable to depression at any stage of their lives came from low social class backgrounds, had been separated from parents before the age of 11, had three or more children under the age of five and lacked a warm, confiding relationship with the husband or male partner. One might speculate that any woman in the situation outlined above would need to be very strong not to be depressed. This influential study ably illustrates the way different factors interact within the coping process to produce apathy and depression. It shows antecedent factors, a high degree of stress and an unsatisfactory support system.

One of the most influential studies of postnatal depression was that of Pitt (1968). He found that ten per cent of a random sample of 305 women were depressed at six weeks post-partum and that a further ten per cent were showing considerable emotional distress. Pitt used the Maudsey Medical Inventory (Eysenck, 1959) during the final trimester to assess personality, and found a marked relationship between high trait anxiety score at that time and depression in the puerperium. He did not, however, find that parity, or the events of pregnancy, labour or delivery had any relationship with the depression. The depressed women expressed feelings of despondency, felt inadequate and were unsure of their ability to cope with the baby. They also complained of marked fatigue and sleep disturbance over and above that which might be expected when caring for a small infant. One of the more disturbing features of this important study was that 43 per cent of the women found to be depressed at six weeks post-partum had not improved when followed up a year later! Pitt concluded that there was a large pool of generally unrecognized distress and depression among postnatal women.

A study by Frommer and O'Shea (1973) considered the effects that maternal deprivation in the mother might have upon her own ability to cope with motherhood. By means of a simple questioning schedule used in antenatal clinics they were able to identify 58 women who had been separated from one or both of their parents before the age of 11 years. Matching this group with 58 controls who had not been separated, they found that women in the index group had a much higher incidence of depression and were much more anxious about their babies, than were those in the control group. They also found that when problems arose in the care of the babies or in their perception of the babies well-being, the separated group became more distressed and anxious than the control group of mothers. Frommer and O'Shea suggested that evidence of separation during childhood could be used by midwives and health visitors to identify vulnerable women. This relationship between maternal deprivation as a child and later depression was also found by Brown and Harris (1978).

The relationships between life-events and postnatal depression can be seen in a number of studies. Paykel et al (1980) in their study of 120 women, found that marital tension acted as a vulnerability factor which produced a negative outcome when another stressful life event or events, e.g. moving house, was also present.

A prospective study of 119 primigravidae (Kumar and Robson, 1978, 1984) used the Eysenck Personality Inventory (EPI) (Eysenck and Eysenck, 1968) to assess the relationship between maternal personality and emotional well-being during pregnancy and at three months post-partum. 16 per cent of the sample were depressed at three months post-partum, and this was associated with marital and family tension, original doubts about continuing with the pregnancy and some history of infertility. They found that high levels of trait anxiety identified by the EPI were associated with depression during the first trimester of pregnancy, but not post-partum depression, and that depressed mothers were more likely to have negative feelings about their three-month-old babies. In their continuation of this study they found that many of the mothers for whom this had been a first experience of depression continued to have psychological problems for up to four years after childbirth.

Cox (1978) studied a group of Ugandan women, and found that 9.7 per cent suffered from postnatal depression, suffering symptoms which were very similar to those described by Pitt (1968) and other researchers. This study and other work, convinced Cox (1986, 1988) of the importance of the sociocultural matrix which surrounds the mother and her family.

This is an argument taken up by Oakley in her study of 55 women (Oakley 1980) from the 28th week of pregnancy until five months post-partum, and clearly illustrated in the work of Stein et al (1989). In Oakley's study depression was defined as a depressed state occurring at any time between discharge from hospital and five months post-partum. Oakley also measured the mother's satisfaction with motherhood via self-reports of feelings about her mothering functions and negative or positive feelings towards the baby. Oakley's study was one of the very few which found any relationship between the events of labour and depression, and one must be cautious of these findings in view of the small sample size. It was found that early postnatal blues were associated with dissatisfaction about the conduct of second stage of labour and with epidural analgesia. Factors associated with depression reflect similar life-stress factors found in other studies; mothers in social classes 4 and 5 suffered depressed moods more frequently, and depression was linked to marital tension and poor housing. Low satisfaction with motherhood was linked to poor support and low self-image.

Social adversity rather than obstetric problems were significant in a study of 483 women (Stein et al ,1989). of whom five per cent were subsequently diagnosed as depressed. Stein and his colleagues focused on two main sets of variables which were expected to have a link with postnatal depression; namely the effect of perinatal complications and factors indicating socioeconomic disadvantage. None of the perinatal factors investigated; length of labour, ante or post-partum haemorrhage, obstetric interventions, perineal tears, and so on, had any relationship with postnatal depression, but social factors of low family income, neither partner being employed and the lack of a confidante were found to be significant.

In an earlier study of the emotional needs of mothers (Ball, 1981), 178 women completed a questionnaire which assessed their degree of satisfaction with their maternity care and about their feelings at six weeks post- partum. Differences in social class, satisfaction with postnatal care, and the mothers self-report of her feelings immediately after delivery were found between the women whose answers revealed high emotional well-being and those who were distressed. Mothers in social class 5 scored lower levels of satisfaction with all aspects of care, and were more often found among the distressed group. Dissatisfaction with postnatal care was associated with marked anxiety about the baby, and complaints about conflicting advice from midwives. There was also some relationship between the mother's reported feelings immediately after the birth and her emotional well-being six weeks later. However, as both reports were completed at six weeks post-partum this may have been due primarily to the mothers emotional state at the time of completion, but it is interesting to note that the same effect was found in the current study even though the assessments were taken at different times in the post-delivery period.

This review of some of the many studies of postnatal depression confirm the view that the coping process was a suitable framework for the research design, and identified factors in the personal and sociocultural matrix of the mother which required to be assessed alongside factors arising from the way in which midwifery care was organized and delivered.

Methods of assessing emotional outcome

One of the problems of this kind of research has been the different types of instruments used to assess emotional well-being post-delivery. Since its development, the 10-point Edinburgh Postnatal Depression Scale (EDPS) (Cox et al ,1987) which was designed purely for the needs of postnatal women, has become the most universal tool for research in this field and in controlled studies of the effect of counselling (Holden et al,, 1989). The EPDS is solely concerned with the mother's emotional state, it does not seek information about satisfaction with motherhood or feelings about the baby. Other studies which predated the development of the EPDS have used a variety of measures. Pitt (1968) used the Maudsey Medical Inventory (Eysenck, 1959) to assess anxiety, and he devised his own depression scale. Kumar and Robson used the Eysenck Personality Inventory (Eysenck and Eysenck, 1968) and the Standardised Psychiatric Interview (Goldberg et al, 1974) to assess depression, as did Stein et al (1989). Paykel et al (1980) used the Raskin Depression Scale (Raskin et al, 1970) together with features drawn from the work of Brown and Harris (1978). Other researchers (Handley et al, 1977, 1980; O'Hara et al, 1982) have used the Beck Depression Inventory (BDI) (Beck et al, 1961).

Maternal-child relationships

The postnatal period does not only mark the end of the pregnancy and labour, but more importantly the beginning (or continuation in more substantial form) of the relationship between the mother and her infant. In the last two or three decades there has been a growing volume of research which has focused upon these relationships.

Bowlby's pioneering work (1951, 1961) on the effects upon the psychological well-being of children of contemporary methods of residential child care led him to the conclusion that a warm, continuing relationship between the child and his mother or permanent mother substitute was essential. The results of his work was to revolutionize attitudes to, and the organization of child care institutions, and to profoundly influence the work of every profession engaged in the care of children.

More recently the work of Klaus and Kennell (1970, 1976, 1982) and their associates (Klaus et al, 1972, 1975; Kennell et al, 1974; Hales et al, 1977) has been a major influence in the care of mothers and their infants. There is convincing evidence that when mothers and babies are encouraged to spend uninterrupted time together immediately after the birth, it has considerable effect upon the mother's pleasure in her child and upon their continuing relationship. Klaus and his colleagues present evidence that the time immediately after birth is particularly important in the establishment of close ties between the mother and her baby. Studies of several groups of mothers found that when left uninterrupted the mother followed a particular pattern of exploring her baby's body. Eye contact has been shown to be particularly important and the work of Leboyer (1975) showed wonderful photographs of the profound gaze in the eyes of a newborn infant. As early as 1977, an editorial in the British Medical Journal (BMJ, 1977) pointed out the significance of these studies, and called for changes in the existing delivery suite and neonatal nurseries in maternity hospitals. Whilst the importance of the first hour or so after delivery was highlighted by their studies, Klaus and Kennell (1982) point out that the relationship between mother and infant is one which grows and develops over the days and weeks, and this can be fostered by easy and regular contact between the child and its parents.

The claim that there is a particularly sensitive period for maternal-infant attachment (Kennell et al, 1975) has been criticised (Dunn and Richards, 1977) and these criticisms are acknowledged (Klaus and Kennell, 1982), but other researchers present results which support this belief (McClellan and Carbianca, 1980). The complexity of these relationships, the factors which influence their development and the difficulties of undertaking research in this field has been reviewed by Seigel (1982). The importance of enhancing good relationships and the problems which arise from difficulties has been highlighted in the research noted earlier which identified the impact of maternal depression upon the emotional and cognitive development of the infant and young child (Murray 1988, Cogill et al, 1986). A number of other studies of the effect of mental illness in mothers are discussed by Melhuish et al (1988).

Klaus and Kennell (1982) suggest that two main groups of factors influence the establishments of early maternal-child relationships. One group relates to maternal antecedent factors: personality; family relationships; cultural influences. The other group of factors arise from the caring environment; attitudes and practices of doctors, midwives and nurses; hospital and care policies, and so on. Such factors are reminiscent of those outlined earlier in the coping process and in studies like those of Frommer and O'Shea (1973). In a Canadian study, Brousard and Hartner (1971) found that mothers whose self-esteem was low were more likely to see their babies as difficult, and were observed to have continuing problems in their relationship with their babies. Lynch et al (1976) found that mothers whose children had been placed on the "at risk" non-accidental injury register suffered from diffuse problems in personal relationships. Retrospective examination of maternity hospital records discovered that the midwives who had cared for these mothers in the immediate postnatal period had observed and recorded that there were difficulties in the way the babies were being nurtured by their mothers. Another study of women who had abused their babies (Rosen and Stein, 1980) found that they had low self-esteem and difficulty in maintaining close relationships. All these studies suggest that some women have particular problems in establishing good and satisfying relationships with their babies, and that the caring environment which surrounds the mother during pregnancy, at the time of birth and during the puerperium may have a unique and strong opportunity to influence the situation for good or ill. Given that antecedent factors are permanent or semi-permanent features of a person's character, the supportive environment which also affects the coping mechanism may be the only factor which can be altered and designed to meet different individual degrees of need.

Support systems and the organization of maternity care

Studies of postnatal depression and maternal-child relationships highlight the many different factors which influence the way women react to motherhood, and the potential influence of the supportive environment. The most important influence is that of the family and close friends, but the caring culture provided by society and its care services also have a role to play (Caplan, 1964, 1969; Caplan and Killilea, 1976). Caplan maintains that the actions and attitudes of professional care givers and the way in which care is organized can be a means of "loading the dice" in favour of a good or bad outcome for individual clients.

Supportive environments and maternity care

This is illustrated in the study by Klaus *et al* (1986) which examined the effect of social support upon maternal and infant morbidity. This randomized controlled study was carried out in a Guatemalan state hospital caring for a population of poor women, who were normally left to undergo labour alone in a busy ward. The study allocated 465 women to one of two groups, the experimental group received support and companionship during labour from a lay Guatemalan woman, in addition to the usual intra-partum care. Those in the control group received the usual care in labour but because of the pressure of work in the hospital did not receive any consistent attention from one person. The lay companions were given the name 'doula', which is the Greek word for women's servant. Although the provision of skilled obstetric care via the hospital had reduced maternal and neonatal mortality in this developing country, its pattern of work had overlooked and disrupted the normal supportive environment in which women gave birth. In providing a lay companion whose function was to provide emotional and physical support, rubbing the mother's back, holding hands, providing explanations and encouragement, the researchers were replacing the kind of female companionship which would have been normal in the family and tribal culture of these women. The results showed clear benefits. Those women who received care from the 'doulas' had significantly fewer perinatal complications with fewer infants needing intensive care, and of those women in either group who had normal labour and delivery, those with the 'doulas' had significantly shorter labours.

The term 'women's servant' is not too far removed from that of midwife 'with woman', and there are some similarities between the role of the 'doula' and the traditional role of the midwife. The findings of this study amply illustrate the benefits of a helpful supportive environment in that particular setting of a busy hospital in a developing country. One must, therefore, be cautious in making direct comparisons between the Guatemalan hospital and those in the United Kingdom, especially in view of the much more relaxed atmosphere, with husbands and other relatives or friends present during labour and at the birth. This study does, however, underline the importance of the supportive environment in reducing stress and improving outcome.

Over the last two or three decades there has been much concern in this country that the opportunities for midwives to provide individual care to their clients has been increasingly eroded, as the maternity services became more centrally organized and hospital-based. Oakley (1994) makes a clear distinction between social support and clinical care or health education, or other aspects of what might be called "professional" care. She maintains that social care is listening, responding, informing when asked, and helping whenever and however appropriate. This personal, interactive companionship and communication which focuses upon the woman and her need at the time is illustrated in Flint's descriptions of ways that midwives can encourage mothers (Flint,1986) and contrasts strongly with the institutionalized and controlling discussions between some midwives, doctors and their clients, which Methven (1989) and Kirkham (1989) observed. These meetings between carers and clients often ignored or did not respond to the mother's questions and fears. All too often, professional staff are unaware of the degree to which their actions are affected by the culture of the organization in which they work.

The maternity services have been the focus of discussion and debate for many years. Until the latter half of the 20th century, most women gave birth at home, receiving what help was available. Before the establishment of domiciliary midwifery services in 1936, working class women found much of the available care to be inadequate and unskilled (Llewellyn Davis, 1979), while for the middle or upper classes some modicum of medical help and nursing care was available (Houldsworth, 1988). After the second world war came the move from home to hospital as the place of birth , there have been many studies and comments on the benefits and hazards of this change (Chard and Richards, 1977; Kitzinger and Davis, 1978; Beech, 1987; Inch, 1989; Chalmers *et al*, 1989; Tew, 1990).

One of the main effects of this move from home to hospital-based births was the disruption of long-standing family and social patterns for support in childbirth, and the exchange of the home bedroom for the sterilized and busy atmosphere of a hospital delivery suite. Kitzinger (1983) describes this experience as being "required to make love, pouring ourselves body and mind, into the full experience of feeling ... in a busy airport concourse, a large railway terminus, a gymnasium or a tiled public lavatory!" It must be said that a great deal has improved since those days. The changes in social attitudes in the 1970s affected hospital practices as the presence of husbands or boyfriends at the birth became commonplace, rather than the rare and grudgingly-granted event it had been before then. Pressures from midwives and consumer groups also brought about many improvements in maternity care.

Making the hospital the normal place for birth had a number of other effects, most particularly the practice of discharging women and babies home to the care of the community midwife within 48 hours or so of the birth. Before this change, it was usual for women delivered in hospital to stay in for at least ten days. Community midwives at that time ran a completely separate service for the women they had delivered in their own home. Transferring women home early in the postnatal period had a number of effects. Arrangements and decisions about the length of stay in hospital were often made during the pregnancy, or imposed by hospital policy, but had to be confirmed by the community midwife. Much time and paper was spent on assessing the suitability of the mother's home for early discharge. If the midwife refused to take a particular mother and her baby home, there were problems and arguments. In hospitals, junior doctors might disrupt the arrangements made, with no valid medical reason and this caused further problems. The timing of 48 hours for early discharge had no physiological basis, but was purely a matter of administrative convenience. The fact that it came about just as breastfeeding was being established was not taken into consideration, nor was the mother's degree of confidence in caring for her new infant.

The sharing of postnatal care led to a number of agreements drawn up between hospital and community services concerning the different tasks which were to be performed by each. Generally if a woman had booked for a 48 hour discharge, the hospital midwives would help in the initiation of feeding and provide care for the baby, but leave the bulk of mothering education to the community midwife. This created a chronological and routinized approach to the amount of care and help a mother received, irrespective of her individual needs. Routine-centred patterns of care and the increasingly rapid turnover of women from postnatal wards made it difficult for midwives to provide sensitive care for individual women, or cater for the needs of inexperienced or anxious mothers (Ball and Stanley, 1984; Laryea, 1984).

It was in order to reduce this increasing fragmentation of care that many schemes such as the Domino system (where a community midwife brings her client in for delivery and takes her home within about six hours after the birth) and team midwifery (Flint and Poulengeris, 1987) were developed. Much of the evidence given to the Winterton Committee (House of Commons, 1992) highlighted the growing concern about the need for changes in the organization of maternity care which would focus more clearly on the needs and wishes of the mother and enable midwives to provide the necessary continuity and consistency of care to women throughout pregnancy, labour and the puerperium. Currell (1990) reviewed many of these issues, illustrating the impact which the organization of a service has upon its care providers and their clients, the difficulties inherent in meeting individual needs within a large care organization. She considered that the answer lies in ensuring a unity rather than continuity of care, arguing that while continuity is concerned with being continuous, the term unity implies oneness of purpose, being formed of parts which make up a complex whole. Providing unity of care means that the service must focus upon the woman rather than the caregiver so that the woman becomes the centre of the service, which is organized to ensure that "all encounters with staff contribute to the whole". Currell quotes from the work of Campbell (1984) who describes nursing/midwifery as skilled companionship. "The good companion is someone who shares freely, but does not impose, allowing others to make their own journey".

Midwives role in reactions to motherhood

The evidence arising from the concepts of the coping process, studies of reactions to motherhood and the formation of maternal-child relationships all identify factors in the woman and her environment which together will influence the emotional outcome. Midwives provide the bulk of care to women and their babies, and are in an unique position to provide individualized, need-focused care, and to bring about those changes in the organization of services which will best promote this quality of care. At best midwives are in a position to enhance and enrich the experience of motherhood, at worst they should be able to avoid causing any extra stress because they do not understand or appreciate the complexity of the many events and processes involved in adjusting to this crucial and life-affected job of being a mother. This then was the purpose behind the research, to study women's reactions to motherhood and discover whether any particular pattern of care provided by midwives or the maternity services as a whole had any significant effect upon the mother's emotional well-being and satisfaction with motherhood six weeks after the birth of the baby.

CHAPTER 4

Undertaking the Research

In view of the issues which arise from a review of the many and varied factors involved in adjusting to motherhood, the question to which the research addressed itself was:

> Given the many internal and external factors which are likely to affect the way women react to the birth of a child, what effect, if any, do the current patterns of postnatal care provided by midwives working in the National Health Service, have upon the way women adjust to the demands of motherhood.

Working hypotheses

1. The emotional response of women to the changes which follow the birth of a child will be affected by their personality and by the quality of the support they receive from family and social support systems.
2. The way in which care is provided by midwives during the postnatal period will influence the emotional response of women to the changes which follow the birth of a child.

Patterns of care at time of the research

The research was conducted in three hospitals during 1980 and 1981. In general, the organization of care was very similar to that of 1994, but a number of practices designed to provide greater continuity of care and control for the mother had not been introduced. The most usual pattern of care was for the woman to be booked for hospital delivery via her general practitioner and community midwife, and antenatal care was shared between the hospital and community services. Communication between these services was maintained via the cooperation card system, and it was rare for women to carry their own records. Birth plans had not been developed, so that the mother's wishes in regard to care in labour may or may not have been explored, and were not usually recorded. Team midwifery did not exist, although community midwives did maintain their specific caseload of mothers and provided some needed consistency of care and care provider. Some services ran Domino systems but these affected only a minority of mothers and midwives. The most usual pattern was for the woman to telephone the hospital when she found herself to be in labour, and to be admitted to the labour ward, where she would receive care from the staff on duty on that particular shift. Many midwives working in labour wards endeavoured to stay with a mother throughout her labour, but this was not a general policy and shift systems and work allocation patterns often made it difficult to achieve this. Postnatal care was very similar to that of today. After delivery, mothers and babies were transferred to the postnatal ward with its separate staff. Here they would receive care, help with establishing infant feeding, and in most cases be transferred home under the care of the community midwife about 48 hours after the birth. Mothers who had obstetric or neonatal complications would remain in hospital care for a longer period. Another feature of 1980 which has largely died out, was the existence of general practitioner maternity units to which many mothers were transferred for extra rest and care before going home. These units were small, often housed in pleasant large houses, and were very popular. Evidence given to the Winterton Committee (House of Commons, 1992) suggested that their demise was regrettable.

The research was designed as a descriptive study of the experiences and reactions of women during childbirth and the first six weeks of their infant's life, as they coped with and adapted to the demands which the birth of their infant made upon them and their families. It was a mainly prospective study in terms of the events of labour and postnatal care and the assessment of emotional well-being in the mother six weeks after delivery, but also contained retrospective elements in the mother's assessment of labour and the postnatal care she had received.

The research method was based upon a descriptive survey methodology described by Oppenheim (1966) as an analytic and relational survey. It was designed to allow statistical analysis by computer.

Descriptive surveys are usually based upon a representative sample of the target population in order that the findings may be generalized to the population as a whole. It was not possible, within the constraints of time and finance, to base this survey upon such a representative sample. Instead, a cohort group of women in late pregnancy were studied who were booked for delivery in one of three maternity hospitals. They were included in the research from approximately the 36th week of pregnancy until six weeks after the birth of the baby.

The target population was defined as pregnant women booked for delivery in Consultant Maternity Hospitals in England during 1981 and 1982. The three hospitals selected were each in a different part of the country. Hospital 1 was a large hospital sited in a cathedral city and serving a wide urban and rural population. Hospital 2 was a smaller hospital in an industrial town in the Midlands, serving mainly a mining and industrial community. Hospital 3 was a professorial unit which had a number of regional sub-specialities and served women from a wide range of other health authorities as well as its own inner city population.

In order to achieve a sample sufficiently large to allow the effects of postnatal care to be differentiated from other factors involved in emotional well-being it was decided to aim for a sample of 100 women in each hospital. The target recruitment number in each hospital was then set at 120 to allow for wastage due to non-response.

Selection of women for the study

Participants were selected from the antenatal records of women who were due to give birth during the three months of the study. In order to avoid a number of extraneous variables which might affect maternal perceptions of pregnancy, birth and puerperium, the following categories of women were excluded from the selection process.

1. Women with a history of infertility leading up to the current pregnancy.
2. Women who had suffered stillbirth or neonatal death in a previous pregnancy; those who had required admission to an antenatal ward before the 36th week of their current pregnancy; women with diabetes or other known medical complications; women with known multiple pregnancy.
3. Women from Asian communities were excluded because of language difficulties and different cultural attitudes. West Indian women who had been born in the United Kingdom were included; those born in the West Indies were excluded.
4. Mothers aged under 16 years of age or over 40 years.
5. Mothers whose babies were to be adopted.

Recruitment

The total number of women recruited and for whom full data were obtained is shown in Table 4.1. It can be seen that a smaller number of women were recruited in hospital 3. This was due to severe weather in the winter of 1981, during which many mothers did not attend the antenatal clinic.

Table 4.1:Numbers of mothers recruited and interviewed, final sample and resource rate

	Hospital 1	*Hospital 2*	*Hospital 3*	*Total Sample*
Mothers recruited	122	127	98	347
Interviewed after delivery	117	119	84	320
Returned post-natal questionnaire	112	104	63	279
Response rate of mothers interviewed after delivery	95.7%	87.3%	75.0%	87.0%

Age groups of participants

The age groups of the women in the final sample were as follows:

- under 20 years 31 (11.1 per cent);
- 21-29 years 164 (58.8 per cent);
- 30-39 years 84 (30.1 per cent).

There was no statistically significant difference in the distribution of age groups across the three hospitals (chi-square = 1.33593 with 4 d.f. P = 0.9553).

Parity of the participants

Of the women, 98 (35.4 per cent) were primigravidae, 118 (42.3 per cent) were having their second baby, 38 (13.6 per cent) were having their third baby, and the remaining 25 (9 per cent) were having a fourth child. One set of twins is included in the final sample; these were born to a primigravid woman of 19 years of age.

Social class and marital status of the participants

There was a wide spread of social class in the sample, as can be seen from Table 4.2. There was a significant difference in the distribution of social class of the sample between the three hospitals (chi-square = 31.08387 with 12 d.f.; P = 0.0019). Hospital 1 had the highest proportion of mothers from social classes 1 and 2, and hospital 3 had the highest proportion of mothers from social class 5.

Of the mothers, 29 were single (10.4 per cent), five were separated or divorced (1.8 per cent) and the majority, 245 (87.8 per cent) were married and living with their spouse.

Table 4.2:Distribution of social class of the sample by hospital

	Social Class									
	1 and 2		3n/m[a]		3m[b]		4 and 5		Unclassified	
	n	%	n	%	n	%	n	%	n	%
Hospital 1	40	52.1	19	48.7	26	38.1	21	24.0	6	54.5
Hospital 2	22	23.5	19	48.7	28	41.2	31	40.0	3	27.3
Hospital 3	23	24.3	1	2.6	14	20.6	22	36.0	2	18.2
Total	85	30.7	39	14.1	68	24.5	74	26.7	11	4.0

[a]   n/m, non-manual
[b]   m, manual
[c]   Two missing cases

Choice of hospitals

The three hospitals were selected because each was operating a slightly different method of organizing postnatal care. In all three, the majority of mothers and babies went home around 48 hours after delivery, and all the hospitals were midwifery training schools.

Hospital 1 had 101 beds, and 4,040 births during 1981. In this district all mothers booked for hospital delivery were visited by their community midwife at least three times during pregnancy, and for at least 28 days after the birth.

Hospital 2 had 52 beds, and 2,600 births during 1981. There was no regular pattern of visiting the mother at home during pregnancy, and mothers were visited daily for at least ten days after delivery. When the midwife considered it necessary the visits were extended beyond ten days and up to 28 days.

Hospital 3 had 149 beds, and 4,500 births during 1981. In this hospital the postnatal wards were said to be operating a patient allocation system which meant that each mother came under the care of a particular midwife. There was, however, no contact between this midwife and the mother before the baby was born and observation of the ward during the study did not find that there was any real allocation of mothers to midwives. As a result of the number of other health districts from which this hospital drew its patients, there was no consistent policy of visiting by community midwives, and the degree of contact between the hospital and community services was extremely variable.

Research design

It would be unrealistic to study the relationship between mothers and midwives in isolation from the many other factors which have been shown to affect postnatal emotional well-being. Accordingly, the research design was based upon the concepts of the coping process and support systems. A number of factors arising from previous research were incorporated in the design in the hope of reducing possible distortion of the results by the presence of potent but unrecognized factors, and in order to compare any results related to midwifery care with those of other studies.

Factors in the research design

The factors included in the design are listed below.

1. Personality of the mother (Pitt, 1968; Kumar and Robson, 1978, 1984; Wilson-Barnett, 1979). This was assessed by the use of the Eysenck Personality Inventory, which provides a measure of anxiety trait and extroversion/introversion.
2. Maternal separation from her own mother before the age of 11 years (Frommer and O'Shea, 1973; Brown and Harris, 1978; Kumar and Robson, 1984).

3.   Life crisis events occurring during the year preceding the birth (Holmes and Rahe, 1967; Paykel, 1980; Kumar and Robson, 1978, 1984). The life-crises included were:
     • death of a close family member;
     • illness/injury of a close family member;
     • changes in marriage/partnership;
     • changes in residence or living conditions;
     • changes in husband's employment;
     • changes in own employment;
     • any other stressful changes reported by the mother.
4.   Time of first holding the baby, time of first feeding the baby, any separation of mother and baby during the stay in hospital (Klaus and Kennell 1970, 1976, 1982).
5.   Mother's reported feelings after the birth (Ball 1981).
6.   Mother's self-image (Broussard and Hartner, 1971; Lynch et al. 1976; Oakley, 1980; Rosen and Stein, 1980).

The research design is illustrated in Figure 4.1.

Data collection from mothers
Data was collected from the mother on three occasions.

1.   Each mother was recruited during a visit to the antenatal clinic at around the 36th week of her pregnancy. During this interview a number of questions were asked about her personal circumstances, and about what she was most looking forward to, or fearing, concerning the impending birth. Most women said that they were most looking forward to 'getting it over with', but a number said they were most looking forward to being a mother. During this interview questions were asked about separation from the woman's own mother before the age of 11, and each woman was asked to complete the Eysenck Personality Inventory before she left the clinic.

2.   Each mother was then visited in hospital within 24-36 hours after the birth of her baby. Before the interview a full record of the events of the labour and delivery was obtained. This interview took place in private at the mother's bedside and allowed for the exploration of a number of issues. First the mother's perceptions of the birth were discussed and four rating scales were completed. These asked the mother to rank a number of questions about:

     • her assessment of the birth as an experience in life as a whole;
     • her experience of labour and delivery compared with her expectation of it;
     • her perception of pain during labour;
     • her recall of her own feelings immediately after the birth.

Fig. 4.1:Model of research design for the study of the emotional needs of mothers during the perinatal and postnatal periods.

Conceptual bases: COPING PROCESS   SUPPORT SYSTEMS
                 (Lazarus, 1966)   (Caplan, 1969)

Antecedent factors (late pregnancy)

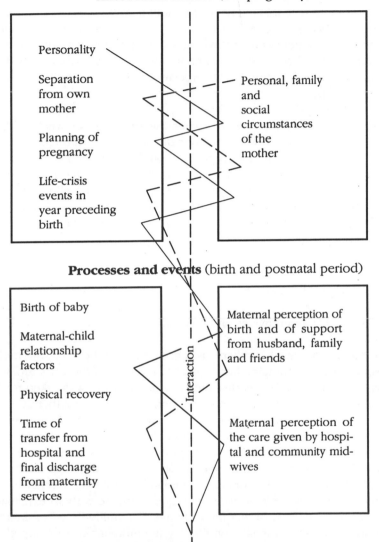

Personality

Separation
from own
mother

Planning of
pregnancy

Life-crisis
events in
year preceding
birth

Personal, family
and
social
circumstances
of the
mother

Processes and events (birth and postnatal period)

Birth of baby

Maternal-child
relationship
factors

Physical recovery

Time of
transfer from
hospital and
final discharge
from maternity
services

Interaction

Maternal perception of
birth and of support
from husband, family
and friends

Maternal perception of
the care given by hospi-
tal and community mid-
wives

Outcome (six weeks after the birth)

Measure of emotional well-being
and satisfaction with motherhood.
Mother's perception of current support from husband, family and
friends.

With the exception of the pain perception scale, all the items were ranked from 1 to 5, with a further category for those women who felt that none of the statements offered adequately expressed her feelings. The pain perception scale was based upon Hayward's (1975) pain scale and the scores ranged from 'the pain was unbearable most of the time' to 'the pain never upset me during labour'.

During the rest of this interview the mother was asked about concurrent life-crisis events affecting her or her family, she was asked to recall the time when she first held and first fed her baby after delivery, and she was asked a number of other questions about the organization of her postnatal care, and the amount of support she expected to receive from her family on her return home.

3.   The mother was next contacted when the baby was six weeks old. At that time she was sent a postal questionnaire which was in three parts. Part 1 asked her to rate a number of items about her care in the hospital postnatal ward. Part 2 asked her to rate the care she had received from the community midwives. Part 3 was a questionnaire about her feelings about herself, the baby and the quality of support she was receiving at the time from her family. The structure of this questionnaire will be discussed more fully later.

Data collection from midwives

Data was obtained from midwives on two occasions.

1.   On the day that each mother was sent home from hospital, the midwife responsible for arranging her transfer to the care of the community midwife was interviewed. During this interview the midwife was asked for her assessment of the physical and emotional state of the mother at the time of discharge, and about her ability to cope with her baby. In a considerable number of cases the midwife arranging the transfer had not had much contact with the mother during the previous few days and made her judgements on the basis of the nursing records. These were also the basis of information sent to the community midwife about each mother.

2.   Each community midwife received a questionnaire with an explanatory letter via the mother on her return home. The midwife was asked to complete the questionnaire on the day the mother was discharged. The community midwife was asked similar questions to those asked of the hospital midwife, and in addition was asked to record the time when the mother was first visited after her return from hospital, and the length of time after the birth during which the mother received care from the community midwifery services.

Copies of all the questionnaires can be found in Appendix I.

During the period of the study in each hospital non-participant observation of the postnatal ward was undertaken and notes kept of the way the wards were organized. The researcher also sat in at a number of shift report sessions, and examined the type of information sent to community midwives and health visitors.

Design, structure and factor analysis of the postnatal questionnaire

As previously stated, this questionnaire was in three parts. Parts 1 and 2 were concerned with the mother's retrospective assessment of the care she received and her feelings during her stay in hospital and during the period when the community midwife was visiting her at home after delivery.

Hospital-based postnatal care

This questionnaire consisted of 16 statements designed to assess:

- mother's self-image during her stay in hospital;
- her perception of infant feeding and the amount of help given;
- whether the mother had felt relaxed in the ward situation and able to rest sufficiently;
- her perception of the support given by midwives.

Postnatal care given at home

This questionnaire consisted of 14 statements designed to assess:

- mother's self-image at that time;
- her perception of her ability in feeding the baby;
- the amount of rest she had and the demands made by her family;
- her perception of the support given by midwives.

Scoring system

All the statements in the postnatal questionnaire were designed to allow a range of five responses, from 'strongly agree' to 'strongly disagree'. These responses were scored from 1 to 5, with the score of 3 being given to a non-committal response of 'neither agree nor disagree' and the highest score to the most favourable response. For example, a positive statement such as 'I felt fit and well soon after my baby was born' would be scored as follows:

- Strongly agree - **Score 5**
- Agree - **Score 4**
- Neither agree nor disagree - **Score 3**
- Disagree - **Score 2**
- Strongly disagree - **Score 1**

On the other hand, a negative statement such as 'I didn't feel well enough to look after my baby' was scored in the opposite direction, so that the most positive response again received the highest score, thus:

- Strongly agree - **Score 1**
- Agree - **Score 2**
- Neither agree nor disagree - S**core 3**
- Disagree - Score 4
- Strongly disagree - Sc**ore 4**

The statements were written in varied forms in order to avoid a response set (Oppenheim, 1966). Two further questions were included. On the hospital-based questionnaire (Part 1) the mother was also asked to indicate whether in retrospect she considered the time spent in hospital had been right for her or not. On the community-care-based questionnaire (Part 2) mothers for whom it was appropriate, were asked how their older child or children had reacted to the advent of the new baby. The answers to these questions were not included in the overall scores on the postnatal statements. In addition, the mothers were invited to add any other comments they wished. The total score for Parts 1 and 2 of the questionnaire was used in a limited way to assess mother's overall reactions. The results of all the questionnaires were subjected to factor analysis and the factor scores which emerged from this process were then used as variables in the analysis. Factor analysis is a statistical technique based upon intercorrelating all the items being investigated with each other, in order to abstract one or more underlying factors which the items have in common (Oppenheim, 1966; Stopher and Meyburg, 1979). The emerging factors are listed in order of their strength and consistency.

Factor analysis

Six factors emerged from the hospital postnatal care questionnaire, and four from the questionnaire about postnatal care at home.

Hospital-based postnatal care

The formation of each factor emerging from the hospital-based questionnaire and the factor loading for each statement after Varimax rotation are listed below.

Factor 1. Feeding support factor

This was formed from the answers to four statements:

Statement	Factor loading
'The midwives and nurses were helpful when I was feeding my baby'	+ 0.83325
'I was helped to feel confident when I was feeding my baby'	+ 0.73999
'The midwives and nurses seemed to understand what help I needed'	+ 0.72584
'I needed more help in feeding my baby than I was given'	+ 0.54348

This factor was quite distinct from factor 5, which reflected the mother's perception of her own abilities and skill when feeding her baby during the early postnatal days in hospital.

Factor 2. Ward atmosphere

These four statements reflect anxiety which might be expressed by any patient in any hospital:

Statement	Factor loading
'I felt homesick and lonely'	+ 0.84173
'It was easy to relax and feel at home'	+ 0.57817
'I felt silly asking questions'	+ 0.56929
'Nobody listened to what I said, they just told me what to do'	+ 0.51631

Factor 3. Physical well-being

These statements formed this factor:

Statement	Factor loading
'I didn't feel well enough to look after my baby'	+ 0.85334
'I felt fit and well soon after my baby was born'	+ 0.82465
'Other mothers seemed to manage better than I did'	+ 0.46431

Factor 4. Rest

This proved to be a most interesting factor in the reactions of mothers to the different postnatal care practices in the different hospitals. It was formed from the following statements:

Statement	Factor loading
'It was easy to get enough rest in the day-time'	+ 0.83651
'I needed more rest at night'	+ 0.62377
'It was easy to relax and feel at home'	+ 0.59795

Factor 5. Self-image in feeding

This factor emerged consistently as quite separate from the feeding support factor. It was formed from the following statements:

Statement	Factor loading
'Feeding my baby was a worry'	+ 0.88433
'I needed more help in feeding my baby than I was given'	+ 0.58542
'Other mothers seemed to manage better than I did'	+ 0.58158

Factor 6. Conflicting advice

This final factor was formed from the following statements:

Statement	Factor loading
'Conflicting advice from midwives was upsetting'	+ 0.83843
'Different midwives gave different advice'	+ 0.81843

Postnatal care at home

The factor analysis of the questionnaire about postnatal care at home produced four factors. The factor formation and the factor loading for each statement in the factor after Varimax rotation are given below:

Factor 1. Midwife support

This factor was concerned with the mother's reaction to the way the midwives cared for her:

Statement	Factor loading
'The midwife seemed to understand what help I needed'	+ 0.86127
'The midwife's visit was a great help'	+ 0.83750
'The midwife always seemed to be in a hurry'	+ 0.67615

Factor 2. Continuity of advice
This factor reflected not only the advice received from midwives and health visitors, but also that given by family and friends:

Statement	Factor loading
'Different midwives gave me different advice'	+ 0.76022
'The health visitor and midwife gave conflicting advice'	+ 0.65232
'There were too many different mid-wives visiting me'	+ 0.64678
'Too many people gave me advice'	+ 0.64188

Factor 3. Rest/family support
These statements formed this factor:

Statement	Factor loading
'The family expected me to do too much'	+ 0.83766
'After I came home it was difficult to get enough rest'	+ 0.75567
'My husband seemed to know what help I needed'	+ 0.63743

Factor 4. Self-confidence
This factor reflects Pitt's description of a mother's confidence in caring for her baby:

Statement	Factor loading
'I felt I couldn't cope on my own'	+ 0.78537
'I felt confident in handling my baby'	+ 0.77457
'I needed more help in feeding my baby than I was given'	+ 0.53812

Design, structure and factor analysis of the emotional well-being and satisfaction with motherhood questionnaire

It must be emphasized that the questionnaire was designed to provide a measure of the mother's self-report of her feelings six weeks after the birth of her infant. It is not an assessment of clinical depression, but it was derived from methods used in other studies and patterned upon the Beck Depression Inventory (BDI).

The BDI (Beck *et al*, 1961) has been found to have a high degree of reliability, and self-evaluation using this inventory produced results which were consistent with independent clinical examination. Pitt (1968) designed a questionnaire to assess postnatal depression that covers much of the same ground. Kumar and Robson (1978) used the Standardised Psychiatric Interview (Goldberg et al , 1974). However, this is designed to be used by psychiatrists trained in its methods, which made it unsuitable for use in the present study.

It was decided to base the questionnaire on the BDI and Pitt's questionnaire. It was not considered realistic to measure emotional well-being in isolation, and statements assessing the mother's satisfaction with motherhood and with the support she was receiving from her family were also included.

Certain items in the BDI were not included, either because they were considered inappropriate or because the same item was dealt with more appropriately in Pitt's questionnaire. For examine, statements in the BDI based upon pessimism or self-punitive wishes including thoughts of death or suicide were thought to be potentially harmful in a questionnaire whose purpose was to explore the feelings of normal mothers.

Assessment of emotional well being

A total of 19 statements were used to assess emotional well-being based on Beck *et al* (1961) and Pitt (1968).

Depression (Pitt) Mood (Beck) Crying spells (Beck)
'Most of the time I feel happy and cheerful'
'I've felt in low spirits since my baby was born'

Dependency (Pitt) Sense of failure (Beck)
'I feel confident about the way I cope'
'I don't like to be left alone'

Anxiety (Pitt): (a) General, (b) Baby
'I worry a lot'

Depersonalization (Pitt): (a) Self, (b) Baby
'Sometimes I feel I am a machine, not a person'
'Sometimes it feels as if the baby doesn't belong to me'

Sleep disturbances (Beck, Pitt)
'I sleep well when the baby will let me'

Irritability (Beck, Pitt)
'I easily get upset if things go wrong'
'I lose my temper more than I used to'

Guilt (Beck, Pitt) Self-hate (Beck)
'I blame myself for problems with the baby'
'If I had more help I would manage better than I do'

Indecisiveness (Beck)
'I find it hard to make up my mind'

Appetite (Beck, Pitt)
'I don't enjoy food the way I used to'

Libido (Beck, Pitt)
'Sex doesn't interest me as much as before'

Work inhibition (Beck) Retardation (Pitt)
'I feel full of energy these days'
'I feel tired and weary'

Body image (Beck) Hypochondriasis (Pitt; also Gruis, 1977)
'Getting my figure back is important to me'

Assessment of satisfaction with motherhood

The statements about the role of mothering and the mother's perception of her infant's response were designed to assess her feelings about the responsibilities of mothering. The statements used are listed below.

- 'The time I spend with my baby is the best part of the day'

- 'I talk to my baby quite a lot'

- 'I feel that my baby knows that I love him/her'

- 'Being a mother is satisfying'

- 'Sometimes I wish I could go away on my own'

- 'Caring for a small baby makes me feel nervous'

- 'I enjoy stroking my baby's skin'

A separate question which was not included in the total sum of scores on satisfaction with motherhood was added to assess further the mother's perception of her infant. This was patterned upon the Neonatal Perception Inventory devised by Broussard and Hartner (1971), and asked the mother to compare her infant with the 'average' baby in such areas as crying spells, feeding and sleeping patterns, and settling down into a routine. There was no suggestion given in the inventory as to what 'average' was, as the criterion upon which it is based is the individual mother's perception of 'average' behaviour.

Assessment of quality of support

These statements were designed to assess the mother's perception of the availability and quality of help provided by family and friends, and her feelings about the amount of help she needed. Thus a statement such as, 'My family and friends are helpful' would measure the degree to which she saw them as helpful, whereas a statement such as, 'Sometimes I feel overwhelmed by all that I have to do' would measure how she felt about her situation irrespective of the help available to her. The statements about the quality of family support are:

- 'I wish someone would tell me I'm doing a good job'

- 'My family and friends are helpful'

- 'Sometimes I feel overwhelmed by all that I have to do'

- 'My husband gives me all the help I need him to give'

- 'If I need help there is always someone I can turn to'

- 'Sometimes I feel lonely and isolated'

Factor analysis

The factor analysis produced seven factors from the 32 statements in the questionnaire. Five factors were centred upon emotional well-being, one on satisfaction with motherhood, and one on family support. The seven factors are listed below with details of the eigenvalues and factor loading:

	Eigen value	% of variance	Cumulative % of variance
Depression/mood factor	7.05457	22.0	22.0
Satisfaction with motherhood factor	2.64876	8.3	30.3
Coping ability factor	1.75662	5.5	35.8
Anxiety	1.58048	4.9	40.7
Family support factor	1.43080	4.5	45.2
Sleep/anxiety	1.26420	4.0	49.2
Self-confidence	1.14572	3.6	52.8

One of the more interesting features of this factor analysis was that the Satisfaction with Motherhood factor emerged so highly, immediately after the depression/mood factor and before factors emerging from other aspects of coping and anxiety. This is particularly significant when one considers how many studies of postnatal depression have concentrated solely upon measuring emotional responses without relating them to the mother's pleasure or satisfaction in motherhood. Later analysis of the data showed quite distinct factors relating to satisfaction with motherhood which were not related to emotional well-being.

The factor formation and the factor loadings for each statement in the factor after Varimax rotation are given below:

Factor 1. Depression/mood

Statement	Factor loading
'I feel full of energy these days'	+ 0.71115
'Most of the time I feel happy and cheerful'	+ 0.64109
'I feel tired and weary'	+ 0.63796
'I've felt in low spirits since my baby was born'	+ 0.62998
'Sex doesn't interest me as much as before'	+ 0.50936
'I easily get upset if things go wrong'	+ 0.47312

Factor 2. Satisfaction with motherhood

Statement	Factor loading
'I feel that my baby knows that I love him/her'	+ 0.74798
'The time I spend with my baby is the best part of the day'	+ 0.65983
'Being a mother is satisfying'	+ 0.65878
'I talk to my baby quite a lot'	+ 0.63023
'I enjoy stroking my baby's skin'	+ 0.48598

Factor 3. Coping ability

Statement	Factor loading
'Sometimes I feel overwhelmed by all that I have to do'	+ 0.65084
'Sometimes I feel I am a machine not a person'	+ 0.61579
'If I had more help I would manage better than I do'	+ 0.58480
'Sometimes I wish I could go away on my own'	+ 0.50075

Factor 4. Anxiety

Statement	Factor loading
'I find it hard to make up my mind'	+ 0.72251
'I blame myself for problems with the baby'	+ 0.59533
'I easily get upset if things go wrong'	+ 0.54585
'I worry a lot'	+ 0.50554

Factor 5. Family support

Statement	Factor loading
'If I need help there is always someone I can turn to'	+ 0.80389
'My family and friends are helpful'	+ 0.76030
'Sometimes I feel lonely and isolated'	+ 0.39468
'My husband gives me all the help I need him to give'	+ 0.39269

Factor 6. Sleep/anxiety

Statement	Factor loading
'I sleep well when the baby will let me'	+ 0.61954
'Sometimes I feel as if the baby doesn't belong to me'	+ 0.58840
'Caring for a small baby makes me feel nervous'	+ 0.57560
'I feel confident about the way I cope'	+ 0.44552
'I don't like to be left alone'	+ 0.36831

This factor appears to be very like the description given by Pitt (1968) of the 'atypical'depression following childbirth. Pitt described the emotionally distressed women in his study as expressing anxiety about the baby and their ability to cope with the baby even though all the babies in his study were thriving.

Factor 7. Self-confidence

Statement	Factor loading
'I don't enjoy food the way I used to'	+ 0.74289
'I wish someone would tell me I'm doing a good job'	+ 0.54473
'Sex doesn't interest me as much as before'	+ 0.39929
'I lose my temper more than I used to'	+ 0.37895

It can be seen that all the original statements derived from either Beck *et al* or Pitt consistently loaded on to the emotional well-being factors (factors 1, 3, 4, 6 and 7). In addition, two statements designed to assess family support and two designed to assess satisfaction with motherhood also loaded on to the emotional well-being factors. These were the statements:

'I wish someone would tell me I'm doing a good job'

'Sometimes I feel overwhelmed by all I have to do'

'Sometimes I wish I could go away on my own'

'Caring for a small baby makes me feel nervous'

The use of the factor scores

A score for each factor was produced by adding together the scores for the mother's response to each of the statements which formed the factor. As was explained earlier, the response to each statement was scored from 1 to 5, and in each case the lowest score indicated the least favourable response. These scores were then used to assess the individual mother's degree of anxiety, satisfaction, and so on, and the group scores for different categories of mothers were also used to compare their responses. An example of a factor score is given below.

Example: Self-confidence factor (postnatal care at home)
This factor was formed from three statements:

'I felt confident in handling my baby' score = 3

'I felt I couldn't cope on my own' score = 2

'I needed more help in feeding my baby than I was given' score = 4

Total factor score = 9

As the highest possible score per statement was 5, then the best possible score for the factor would be 15, and the lowest would be 3. By grouping women together under various headings, e.g. age, social class, degree of emotional well-being, it was possible to compare the mean factor scores for each group and discover whether there were any significant differences. This was done for all the factors which emerged from the analysis and these factor scores were used as the main variables in the research.

Emotional well-being/satisfaction with motherhood and family support factor scores

The emotional well-being questionnaire was designed to give an overall measure of the emotional state of the mother six weeks after the birth of her baby. Whilst it would have been interesting to compare different aspects of the factors for emotional well-being which were produced, it was decided to use the scores of the 23 statements which formed the five emotional well-being factors (factors 1, 3, 4, 6 and 7) to produce a total score which would provide a measure of the emotional well-being of the mother. Three of the emotional well-being statements appear more than once in the formation of the emotional well-being factors, but their scores were used only once in the combination of statement scores which made up the total emotional well-being score.

Summary of the data collected

The research collected a wealth of information about the mothers in the sample. As well as obtaining information on the personal characteristics of the mothers, life-stress events, their family situations and events of the labour, delivery and postnatal care, the data also produced a series of factor scores which assessed the outcome in terms of the mother's perception of the birth, her satisfaction with the postnatal care she had received, and her emotional well-being, perception of family support and her satisfaction with motherhood six weeks after the birth.

Extra information from the mothers

Each mother was invited to add further comments about any aspect of her postnatal care, or about her feelings at the time when she completed the postnatal questionnaire. This proved very useful as quite a number of the mothers used this facility to expand on some of their answers.

CHAPTER 5

Some Details about the Mothers, their Birth Experiences and Postnatal Care they Received

Many of the mothers involved in the study said that they had enjoyed taking part and found it refreshing that their impressions and views of the midwifery service were being sought.

The outcome of the birth experience in terms of the mother's emotional well-being will be discussed in the following chapters. This chapter will concentrate on the personal details of the mothers, the events of labour and the postnatal care received.

Personal details of the mothers

As described in the preceding chapter, 58.8 per cent of the mothers were aged between 20 and 29 years, 35.4 per cent were primigravidae and 42.3 per cent were having their second child. Of the mothers, 124 (44.4 per cent) came from social classes 1, 2 and 3 non-manual, 142 (50.9 per cent) from social classes 3 manual, 4 and 5, and the remaining 11 mothers were unclassified as regards social class. (No details were obtained for two mothers.)

Planning of the pregnancy

Of the mothers, 188 (67.4 per cent) said that they had planned the pregnancy. There were no significant differences in the parity or social class of women who had planned the pregnancy and those who had not, but only 40 per cent of women under 21 years of age had planned the pregnancy compared with 71 per cent of those over 21 years. It had originally been decided to ask this question during the antenatal interview, but many of the participants said they would prefer to discuss this matter after the baby was safely born, and it was therefore included in the post-labour interview. Some mothers said that they had a fear of 'ill wishing' the baby if they talked about its planning before it was born. It was found that whether the pregnancy was planned or not had no direct link with the subsequent emotional status of the mother.

Reported separation from own mother

A total of 33 women (12 per cent) reported that they had been separated from their own mother for a period of at least three months before the age of 11 years. In most cases this was due to the death of the mother or the breakdown of the parents' marriage when the mother had relinquished the care of her daughter and had sporadic or no further contact. One woman included in this category said that she had been emotionally separated from her mother all her life!

Life-crisis events

A surprising number of women reported life-crisis events during the year of the pregnancy. Sixty-one (22 per cent) had suffered the death of a close family member, and one woman had been widowed during her pregnancy. She had nursed her husband until his death from Hodgkin's disease four months before their second child was born. Although she was still grieving the loss of her husband, she did not subsequently suffer from postnatal emotional distress.

Moving house or having major structural alterations to the house was frequently reported. Altogether 112 women (40 per cent) moved house either during pregnancy or within six weeks of the infant's birth, or were still in the throes of major alterations at the time the baby was born.

Ninety women (32 per cent) reported changes in their husband's employment during the pregnancy, 48 women (17 per cent) were on maternity leave from their jobs, and a further 89 (32 per cent) had given up a job entirely as a result of the pregnancy.

Thirty-seven women (13 per cent) had either married or begun living with their male partners during the pregnancy.

During the post-labour interview each woman was asked whether there were any other events or situations apart from those listed above which had caused stress during the pregnancy. Marital or family tension was reported by 52 women (19 per cent), and 26 (9 per cent) said that they were finding it very difficult to adjust to giving up work.

Labour and delivery

Categories of labour

Labour was classified into three categories.

1. *Spontaneous labour* was defined as one which began spontaneously and continued without any augmentation until completion - 123 women (44.1 per cent) had a spontaneous labour.

2.   *Induced labour* was defined as labour which was artificially induced and then continued without further assistance or was augmented by intravenous Syntocinon until completion - 97 women (34.8 per cent) had induced labour.

3.   *Active management of labour* fell into two sub-groups: delivery by caesarean section and labours that began spontaneously but were then augmented by intravenous Syntocinon. Of the women, 58 (20.8 per cent) fell into the active management category, of whom 29 had a caesarean section and 29 an augmented labour ending in vaginal delivery. Of the caesarean sections 16 were elective and 13 were emergency procedures.

Delivery

A normal delivery was had by 195 women (70.1 per cent), 50 (17.9 per cent) had a forceps delivery, four (1.4 per cent) had a breech delivery and 29 women (10.4 per cent) had a caesarean section. (No information was obtained for one women.)

Length of labour and pain relief

The mean average length of labour was seven hours, with 70 per cent of the mothers having a labour of eight hours or less. During labour, 17 mothers did not use any form of pain relief and 36 did not have any sedation during the first stage but used nitrous oxide and oxygen (Entonox) for the second stage.

Of the mothers, 142 (51 per cent) were given pethidine during labour and 66 (24 per cent) had an epidural. A general anaesthetic was given to 16 women (six per cent) undergoing elective caesarean section.

Episiotomy

An episiotomy was performed on 132 women (47 per cent), 51 (18 per cent) had a perineal tear, seven (two per cent) had a perineal tear in addition to an episiotomy and 88 women (32 per cent) had intact perinea.

Third stage

The third stage of labour was normal for 257 women (92.4 per cent). Of the remaining 22 women, 12 had a post-partum haemorrhage, nine had a retained placenta and one had a retained placenta which was accompanied by a post-partum haemorrhage. (Note: details of labour and delivery were missing for one case.)

Husband's presence

All the hospitals made it possible for the mother to have her husband, male partner, or other helper of her choice with her during labour and delivery. In hospitals 1 and 3 this facility extended to the husband being present during caesarean section under epidural analgesia. In 1980 this was a comparatively rare occurrence for most hospitals.

Altogether 184 women (66 per cent) were accompanied by husband or some other helper during labour. It is not known how many of the women who were alone might have received continous support from a midwife or student.

The babies

The sex distribution of the babies was even, with 140 boys and 140 girls being born. This number includes one set of undiagnosed twins (one boy and one girl) born to a 20-year-old primigravida.

All the babies were rated by the Apgar score at one minute after birth, 212 babies (76 per cent) rated 8 or more at minute; nine babies (three per cent) were transferred to the special care baby unit after delivery. Most of these babies were returned to their mothers in the postnatal ward within 24 hours, and all of them were with their mothers by the fifth postnatal day. Neonatal problems, therefore, did not form a significant issue in the experience of the mothers in the sample.

Maternal contact with the baby after birth

Although the work of Klaus and Kennell was comparatively well-known in 1980, practices in delivery suites were very variable, and this is shown in the results. All the hospitals had written policies which required that the baby be given to the mother to hold immediately after birth and that mothers intending to breastfeed should be encouraged to suckle their babies. When the mothers were asked about this event, 191 (68.5 per cent) said that they held their baby immediately after birth, and a further 51 (18.3 per cent) said that although they did not hold their baby immediately they held him or her during the first hour after birth. Of the remaining 37 mothers, 16 (5.7 per cent) held their babies within four hours, nine (3.2 per cent) within four to eight hours, and 12 (4.3 per cent) did not hold their babies until more than eight hours had elapsed. Most of these incidences were due to the administration of a general anaesthetic.

Results were even more disappointing for mothers who wished to feed their baby after birth. Only 40.5 per cent of the total sample were given an opportunity to feed their baby in the labour ward. Of these mothers 85 per cent breastfed and 15 per cent bottlefed their babies. In spite of the hospital policies which encouraged mothers to suckle their babies, only 58 per cent of those who intended to breastfeed were able to do so. Later analysis showed that this was a significant factor in the mothers eventual satisfaction with motherhood.

The mother's perception of labour and the birth of the baby

The scores given on the four rating scales designed to record the mother's perception of her labour and the birth produced some interesting results in view of the arguments which have raged in recent years about the management of birth in hospital.

Each mother was visited in the postnatal ward within 24-36 hours of the birth of her baby. The interviewer had familiarized herself with the details of labour and delivery contained in the obstetric records and after greeting the mother and admiring the baby, the interview usually began with the remark "Well, what was labour like?" This led to a discussion during which the rating scales were completed.

Care received during labour

Almost without exception the mothers were full of praise for the care they had received during labour, and two particular facets of care emerged as having been most helpful.

The first was that one particular midwife, student midwife or in some cases medical student had been personally responsible for the mother's care throughout labour and the delivery, and it was frequently remarked that this had involved that person in staying with the mother after their shift had finished in order to complete the delivery. The mother, her husband and the midwife had used first names, and the picture which emerged was that where the mother felt a personal commitment to her and to her needs by the midwife or student, this had created a strong feeling of security and satisfaction.

These reports closely resemble those described in Shields' (1978) study of nursing care and labour and patients maternal satisfaction. Shields interviewed 80 mothers following delivery; each described the care she had received and rated her level of satisfaction with particular aspects of that care. Mothers described the most helpful aspect of care as the nurses sensitivity to their needs - nurses whose activity and attention in the labour ward were centred upon the mother and her partner and not 'just present in the room'. This sensitivity and attention was rated more highly then the degree of professional competence which the nurse had displayed. This is very interesting in view of the 'doula' study mentioned earlier (Klaus *et al*, 1986) where support from lay women had such a noted impact.

The other aspect of care which drew favourable remarks was that in each of the three hospitals the mother had been carefully consulted about the use of drugs in labour and about any procedure which had been necessary. This approach to joint decision-making had been appreciated by most of the mothers, though some said that they felt the doctor or midwife should have made the decision. This latter group of women felt that they did not want the responsibility of making the decision and were happy to give it to their attendants. Niven (1994) found similar attitudes in her study of the midwife's role on helping a woman cope with labour pain. Out of 26 women who "trusted the staff", 21 were satisfied with their care and had significantly lower levels of pain on some of the recorded measures.

The overriding impression was that the quality of the relationship between the mother and her attendants led to a high degree of mutual respect and trust. Perhaps this is one of the reasons why the results of the labour perception rating scales do not substantiate the claims of certain pressure groups that any interference in the natural progression of labour inevitably produces dissatisfaction with the experience of birth. The results do underline, though, the strongly expressed need for each woman to be treated as a valued individual and to be involved in the decision-making process. They also indicate that some women prefer to give the responsibility for decisions to their attendants; that opinion also should be recognized and valued.

The rating scale results

All the mothers completed these scales even though those who had had an elective caesarean section had not experienced labour. These women often remarked that their 'labour pains' came after the birth, and related their answers to the way they felt on the first day after delivery. On each of the questions there were some mothers who felt that they could not express their feelings fully and that none of the responses adequately reflected how they felt. The results of the birth/labour rating scales are discussed below, and further details of the scores analysed by various maternal and labour factors are shown in Tables 5.1, 5.2 and 5.3.

Table 5.1:Mother's scores on labour perception scales classiified by age and social class (Kruskall-Wallis one-way analysis of variance corrected for ties)

Variable	n	Birth experience (mean rank score)	Expectation of labour (mean rank score)	Feelings after delivery (mean rank score)
(a) Age of mother				
17-20 years	31	143.8	141.9	153.0
21-29 years	161	139.0	138.4	130.8
30-39 years	84	135.6	137.5	147.8
		$x^2 = 0.2797, P = 0.8695$	$x^2 = 0.0724, P = 0.9664$	$x^2 = 3.9226, P = 0.1409$
(b) Social Class				
1	15	169.3	151.5	156.3
2	70	139.3	141.4	139.0
3 non-manual	38	163.3	145.0	141.8
3 manual	67	126.6	135.4	133.8
4	51	129.3	128.3	137.9
5	22	121.3	111.7	111.3
Unclassified	11	121.3	166.4	160.5
		$x^2 =10.2568, P = 0.1142$	$x^2 = 5.0993, P = 0.5311$	$x^2 = 4.7913, P = 0.5708$

Table 5.2: Mothers' scores on labour perception scales classified by type of labour and delivery (Kruskall-Wallis one-way analysis of variance corrected for ties)

Variable	n	Birth experience (mean rank score)	Expectation of labour (mean rank score)	Feelings after delivery (mean rank score)
(a) Type of labour				
Spontaneous	121	137.5	146.7	131.6
Induced	97	139.0	123.3	148.4
Active Management	58	139.7	146.8	136.3
		$x^2 = 0.0409,$	$x^2 = 5.6700$	$x^2 = 2.6064$
		$P = 0.9798$	$P = 0.0587$	$P = 0.2717$
(b) Type of delivery				
Normal	194	142.5	142.5	137.7
Forceps	49	126.2	114.1	133.1
Breech	4	192.5	158.6	161.8
Caesarian Section	29	121.6	150.0	149.8
		$x^2 = 4.8643,$	$x^2 = 6.2598,$	$x^2 = 1.2556,$
		$P = 0.1820$	$P = 0.0990$	$P = 0.7397$

Table 5.3:Mothers' scores on labour perception scales classified by parity and whether the baby was fed in the first hour after birth (Mann-Whitney U test corrected for ties)

Variable	n	Birth experience (mean rank score)	Expectation of labour (mean rank score)	Feelings after delivery (mean rank score)
(a)Parity				
Primigravidae	96	135.2	138.8	141.8
Multiparae	179	138.7	136.8	135.2
		$Z = 0.3645, P = 0.7148$	$Z = 0.2089, P = 0.8345$	$Z= 0.6870, P = 0.4921$
(b)Feeding of baby in first hour				
Fed baby	112	155.2	148.0	151.3
Did not feed baby	164	127.1	132.0	129.8
		$Z = 3.0193, P = 0.0025$	$Z = 1.6822, P = 0.0925$	$Z= 2.2760, P = 0.0228$

Birth as a life experience

- 4 mothers (1.4 per cent) said that the birth was the worst experience of their life
- 15 mothers (5.4 per cent) said that it had been a bad experience
- 103 mothers (36.9 per cent) said that it had been an important experience both good and bad
- 68 mothers (24.4 per cent) said that it had been a good experience
- 76 mothers (27.2 per cent) said it had been the best experience of their life
- 13 mothers (4.7 per cent) did not answer

Thus, just over half the sample recorded that the birth had been a good or best experience. If the scores for each statement are collated then the mean score for the total sample is 3.83, well above the middle of the possible range from worst (score of 1) to best experience (score of 5).

Mothers' experience of labour and delivery compared with their expectations of it

- 26 mothers (9.3 per cent) said that the experience had been much better than they had expected
- 84 mothers (30.1 per cent) said that it had been better than expected
- 61 mothers (21.9 per cent) said that it had been as they had expected it would be
- 49 mothers (17.6 per cent) said that the experience was worse than they had expected
- 30 mothers (13.9 per cent) said that it had been much worse than they had expected
- 20 mothers (7.2 per cent) did not answer

There is a wider set of responses here, and this is reflected in a mean score of 3.01 for the total sample.

Mothers' reported feelings immediately after the baby was born

This emerged as a most interesting set of scores. Earlier work had found a relationship between mothers reported feelings after the birth and her subsequent emotional well-being six weeks later (Ball, 1981). A similar relationship was found in this study and will be discussed further in a subsequent chapter. It should be noted the way women rated birth experience was not directly related to their feelings after the birth. Thus many women who felt that the birth had been a bad experience felt very happy once the baby was born. Most of the women in the sample expressed good feelings after the birth.

- 71 mothers (25.4 per cent) said that they were gloriously happy
- 83 mothers (29.7 per cent) said that they felt tired but happy
- 82 mothers (29.4 per cent) said that they felt relieved
- 19 mothers (6.8 per cent) said that they felt too tired to care
- 6 mothers (2.2 per cent) said that they felt disappointed, and this was mainly due to the sex of the baby
- 18 mothers (6.5 per cent) did not answer

The mothers' scores shown above were not found to be significantly related to age, parity or social class, nor to the type of labour and delivery. The mean score for the whole sample was 3.76 which illustrates the positive nature of most of the responses.

Mothers who fed their babies within the first hour after delivery rated the birth experience more highly than those who did not feed their babies, and they also rated their feelings after the birth more highly than other mothers. This raises the question, 'Which is the chicken and which is the egg?' Was the mother's remembrance of the birth richer because she felt happy? Later analysis revealed that whether a mother fed her baby or not was related closely to her choice of feeding methods, her age and her parity and not to the type of labour or delivery, nor to whether she needed perineal suturing after delivery. These results will be discussed more fully later in relation to the mother's satisfaction with motherhood when the baby was six weeks old.

Table 5.4:Mothers' scores on pain in labour scale classified by parity, length of labour and type of delivery

	Variable	Pain perception	
		n	Mean rank score
(a)	*Parity*		
	Primigravidae	94	115.3
	Multiparae	174	144.9
	Mann-Whitney U test: z = -3.0202, P = 0.0025		
(b)	*Length of labour*		
	4 hours or less	73	134.5
	5-8 hours	105	132.1
	9-13 hours	55	115.7
	13-20 hours	18	87.4
	Kruskall-Wallis test: x^2 = 8.117, P = 0.0438		
(c)	*Type of Delivery*		
	Normal	194	137.2
	Forceps	48	110.1
	Breech	4	189.0
	Caesarian section	24	164.1
	Kruskall-Wallis test: x^2 = 10.5174, P = 0.0146		

Scores on pain in labour

Perhaps it is not surprising to find that the mother's retrospective perception of pain in labour was closely related to the pattern of relief she had used, her parity, and to the length of the labour.

Primigravid women scored significantly lower scores (i.e. more pain experienced) than did multiparae (P = 0.002), and parity is also reflected in scores of those who had a longer labour (P=0.04) and those who had a forceps delivery (P = 0.01) (see Table 5.4).

The highest scores (i.e. indicating those who had not been upset by pain in labour) were those of 16 mothers who used no means of pain relief, and the next highest were those of the 40 women who had an elective epidural, closely followed by those who used only Entonox during the final stages of their labour. The 138 women who received pethidine during labour scored significantly lower scores, and the lowest of all came from those who had been given an emergency epidural after first having pethidine (P = 0.0001).

It should be noted that this was not a controlled trial and that many other factors which would have affected the perception and degree of pain were not recorded. The details of these results can be seen in Table 5.5.

Table 5.5:Mothers' scores on the pain in labour scale classified by method of pain relief used

Method of pain relief	Pain perception	
	n	Mean rank score
Epidural only	40	148.5
Epidural + sedation	24	91.1
Epidural ± Entonox	138	125.8
Entonox only	36	140.6
No pain relief	16	209.2
General anaesthetic[a]	14	154.0

Kruskall-Wallis test:
x^2 = 27.1805, P = 0.0001

a   Applied to pain following anaesthetic

Mothers' opinions about home versus hospital delivery

After all the details of the labour had been discussed, each mother was asked whether, in the light of the events of labour and delivery, she would have preferred the baby to have been born at home. A total of 28 mothers (10.1 per cent) said that they would have preferred a home delivery.

Postnatal care in hospital

The organization of postnatal care in hospital

The observed organization of the postnatal wards was remarkably similar in all three maternity hospitals. All the wards operated on a routine, task-based pattern of care which was mainly determined by the expected time that each mother would spend in the hospital after the birth of the baby.

The progress of care and helping the mother to gain skill and confidence in caring for her baby was arranged on a chronological basis. Mothers who had planned to go home within three days of the birth were not usually shown how to bath their babies whilst in hospital, but it was expected that this would be undertaken by the community midwife.

Supervision of infant care

In each hospital there was a routine pattern of care. On the first day of the baby's life the mothers were shown how to change a nappy, clean the baby's bottom and wash his or her face. She was expected to undertake this care for her baby from then on. On the second day mothers washed their babies, changed nappies and cot linen and fed their babies on demand, with the nursing staff giving support when asked. If the mother was not going home on the third day after delivery she undertook the daily bathing of her baby after a member of staff had demonstrated the correct technique to her. This regime did not appear to make any allowance for the age, parity or physical condition of the mother, who was expected to undertake a chronological progression of feeding and infant care.

One of the results of this routine approach was that mothers who had a painful perineum bathed their babies on the third postnatal day even though sitting on a chair was uncomfortable. For the same reason pain from the perineum was also a problem for mothers who were breastfeeding.

The daily toilet care of the babies took place during the morning period and was mainly supervised by nursing auxiliaries, nursery nurses or junior student midwives. The supervision was allocated to staff on a task allocation basis. Thus a nursery nurse or student midwife might be told to 'see to all the baby baths'. The midwives concentrated on the physical assessment of the mother and discussion with her of the baby's feeding progress. It was not unusual to see a midwife carrying out her daily examination of the mother whilst the baby was being bathed in the nursery.

Division of care

Doctors tended to visit the wards most frequently during the morning shift and this diverted the midwife from the care of the mothers. Doctors also divided the care of the mother and baby, with obstetric housemen concerning themselves mainly with the physical care of the mother, and the paediatric housemen focusing on the care and well-being of the baby.

This fragmentation of care was reflected in the nursing records and reports. Although the nursery nurse or student midwife had supervised the care of the baby and recorded it in the notes she did not normally contribute to any report about the mother's level of skill or confidence in caring for the baby.

Hospital 3 had been included in the study because it claimed to be operating patient-centred care, but the pattern observed was for the mothers in each 'half' of the ward to be allocated to a particular midwife or student midwife for the morning shift. On the following day, although the same staff might be on duty, the allocation did not follow the same pattern but was likely to change according to the attitude of the midwife in charge of the wards. The allocation of staff to patients which had operated on one day did not form a basis for the allocation next morning.

The layout of the ward also affected the pattern of care. In hospital 2, which had Nightingale-type wards, there were very few occasions when nursing staff were not present in the wards, carrying out various tasks or talking to the mother. In the other two hospitals, which had hour-bedded rooms grouped around a central nurses' station, there were considerable periods of time when no nursing staff were to be seen in any of the four-bedded rooms. They tended to go into a room in order to carry out a particular task and then to group themselves in the office, at the central nurses' station, or in the nursery. This meant that there was much less natural interaction between mothers and nursing staff, and mothers were the main initiators of contact with midwives. This was particularly marked in hospital 3 because of the single corridor arrangement of the ward. The lack of windows in the corridor walls of the four-bedded rooms of hospital 3 made it difficult for the mothers to see staff moving from one room to another along the intervening corridor.

Supervision of infant feeding

The mothers were supervised when breastfeeding on the first day after delivery. After the first day supervision was given as required and mothers were expected to feed their babies on demand, filling in a record of the feeds on a chart which was checked from time to time by the nursing staff.

Observation of this system revealed very few occasions when the midwife checked that the length of time the mother said that the infant had been breastfed really corresponded to the amount of time the child had sucked at the breast. Mothers were given advice and encouragement by midwives, but their approach to the feeding of their infants was not normally supervised after the first or second day unless they had been noted as having some difficulty. The advice given to mothers was varied and hardly ever recorded in detail in the nursing record. Instead, terms such as 'needs support' were used with no indication of the type of help needed or offered. Similarly, terms such as 'feeding well' were used to indicate babies of mothers who were seen as needing little or no further supervision. Breastfeeding primiparae received more support in feeding than multiparous women, but primiparae who were bottlefeeding were not given any more supervision than other mothers.

Mothers who bottlefed their babies were not usually supervised, but instructed to feed their babies at least every four hours and write the amount of feed taken on the feeding chart. Very little advice as to the amount of feed required was given. In the main bottlefeeding mothers were given particular advice or supervision only when the baby was considered to be taking too little food or when vomiting had occurred.

The research sample included seven mothers who could not read or write competently. These women overcame the problems of the feeding chart by asking other mothers, or on a number of occasions the author, to fill in the chart on their behalf. At the time when these mothers were discharged from the hospital the midwife arranging for their discharge was asked whether she had realized that the mother could not read or write. With the exception of one mother, who was a gypsy and well-known to the staff, the midwives had not been aware of the mothers' difficulties. Each of these women was bottlefeeding, four were primigravidae, and all had been given written instructions about how to mix the baby's feed, about postnatal exercises, and about postnatal follow-up visits!

Pattern of infant feeding

At the time when the mothers were transferred from hospital postnatal care to either their own homes or to a GP maternity unit the pattern of infant feeding was as listed below.

- Breastfeeding - 161 mothers (57.7 per cent)
- Bottlefeeding - 93 mothers (33.3 per cent)
- Breastfeeding and complementary bottlefeeds - 19 mothers (6.8 per cent)
- Missing information - 6 mothers (2.2 per cent)

At the time when the mothers were discharged from the care of the community midwife the feeding pattern was as follows.

- Breastfeeding - 113 mothers (40.5 per cent)
- Bottlefeeding - 108 mothers (38.7 per cent)
- Breastfeeding and complementary bottlefeeds - 14 mothers (5 per cent)
- Missing information * - 44 mothers (15.8 per cent)

* Due to the amount of missing information it is not possible to draw conclusions about the success or failure of breastfeeding.

It was noted by the hospital midwives that 54 mothers (19.3 per cent) were distressed and anxious about the feeding of their babies. Of these mothers 32 were breastfeeding and 22 were bottlefeeding. Observations of the ward patterns and discussions with the ward sisters did not reveal any system of assessing or planning postnatal care on an individual basis (apart from the decision about the length of time that the mother was likely to spend on the postnatal ward) except when some particular problem had been identified.

Rooming-in patterns

The policies for the rooming-in of mothers and babies in hospitals 1 and 3 were the same. Mothers had their babies by their bedside throughout the day and night from the second night after delivery. In some cases it was noted from observation and mothers' comments that the babies were left with their mothers at night from the day of delivery. The members of the night staff were discouraged from removing babies from their mothers' bedsides at night.

In hospital 2 the pattern was different, and the reason given was the cramped space available in the Nightingale-type wards. In this hospital the babies were taken to the nursery at night and brought to the mothers for feeding during the first two nights after delivery and thereafter according to the mothers' wishes. Most of the mothers went home on the third day after delivery and it was found that those who stayed longer mainly preferred their babies to go into the nursery at night.

Midwives' perceptions of the mother during postnatal care in hospital

Physical well-being

The hospital midwives reported that 218 mothers (78.1 per cent) had made a good physical recovery at the time they were transferred home. In view of the very short time which elapsed between the birth of the baby and the transfer home, this was taken to mean that the physical recovery of the mother from the trauma of the birth was progressing normally.

The assessment of physical recovery also tended to have its own ritual. In all three hospitals the midwife's arrangements for transfer home had to be endorsed by a physical examination of the mother by a junior hospital doctor. This usually took the form of fundal palpation and an examination of the perineum, with little or no reference to the baby's progress or the mother's wishes about her transfer home. This 'medical' approach tended to reinforce the attitude in some families that transfer from hospital meant that physical recovery was complete and that the mother could therefore assume her family responsibilities. It was not uncommon for a junior doctor to pronounce the mother fit for discharge only to find that the midwife had a good reason to recommend a longer stay in hospital (to enable the mother to rest or to acquire more confidence in caring for her baby, or because the community midwife had recommended it). In such cases it was often possible to come to a mutually satisfactory arrangement between the mother and the midwife, but there were also times of conflict and distress caused by such an approach which suggested that the only criterion for discharge was physical.

Emotional needs

During the interview of the hospital midwives, a number of questions were asked about the midwife's perception of the emotional status of each individual mother. The midwives described 218 mothers (78.1 per cent) as appearing 'very happy' or 'placid' during their stay in hospital, 30 (10.8 per cent) as showing a 'mixture of moods', ten (3.6 per cent) as 'withdrawn' and seven (2.5 per cent) as 'distressed'. No opinion was given for 14 mothers (five per cent). When asked in a further question whether the mother had suffered from the 'third day blues' or any other form of emotional distress only three mothers were considered to have had 'the blues' whilst 40 were said to have been distressed for other reasons, the main one of which was physical discomfort.

These reports are surprising in view of the fact that during a separate part of the interview the midwives were asked about certain symptoms of emotional distress which had been seen to affect the mothers during their stay in hospital. In answering this question the midwives cited 60 mothers as having wept during their stay, 41 mothers as having some degree of sleep disturbance, 37 to have shown signs of undue fatigue, eight to have had a poor appetite, and 11 to have shown irritability!

It would appear that the midwives thought that some degree of emotional distress was 'normal' for postnatal women and did not consider this conflicted with their earlier assessment that 78.1 per cent were 'happy' or 'placid'. This is borne out by the comments received from one mother who said 'all the midwives I have talked to say that this survey is a waste of time because all mothers get depressed and there's nothing to be done about it!'

This assumption meant that very little attention was paid to the emotional state of the mother when the arrangements for transfer home were made. It also meant that symptoms of emotional distress were not communicated to the community midwife.

The midwives seemed to be more sensitive to the feelings of mothers when the distress related to difficulties with feeding the baby, 54 mothers (19.4 per cent) were seen to be distressed about the feeding of their babies. Of these 30 were breastfeeding and 24 were bottlefeeding. A high proportion of the breastfeeding women who were reported as being distressed changed from breast to bottlefeeding in the hospital.

Later analysis did not reveal any significant difference in the age, parity or social class of the mothers who were reported as showing symptoms of emotional distress, the 'third day blues', or distress in feeding.

Transfer home and postnatal care in the community

Planned transfer home

All the hospitals had a policy whereby the community midwife was asked to visit the mother at home during pregnancy and assess the length of time she was likely to need to spend in the hospital after delivery. The criteria for assessment were usually the condition of the mother's home and the amount of help she might expect from her family. The assessment was then recorded in the mother's obstetric notes and used as a basis for planning the length of postnatal care in hospital. It was rare to see the length of stay in hospital discussed with the mother after the birth of her baby, and decisions made during pregnancy did not appear to be changed in the light of the events of labour or delivery, or when the mother's home circumstances had changed since the assessment had been done.

Hospital 1 had a policy for the community midwife to visit the mother on three occasions during pregnancy and to make the final assessment approximately four weeks before the expected date of confinement.

During the period of the study in hospital 2 an area of disagreement arose between the hospital and community services and the policy of antenatal assessment at home was not being followed. The community midwives were either not sending in a recommendation at all, or were assessing the mother's needs without visiting her home. In hospital 3 there was a policy for mothers' needs to be assessed by the community midwife and for her to recommend the time of transfer home.

The effectiveness of the policies can be seen in Table 5.6, which shows that although 95 per cent of the mothers in hospital 1 had been visited by a community midwife, the percentage was much lower in the other two hospitals.

Table 5.6:Difference between hospitals in antenatal visiting by community midwives[a]

Hospital	The midwife visited		The midwife did not visit	
	n	%	n	%
1	107	95.5	5	4.5
2	28	26.4	78	73.6
3	36	58.1	26	41.9

$x^2 = 102.47593$, 2d.f.; $P = 0.0001$

a   As reported by mothers

Although only 28 mothers in hospital 2 had been visited, the community midwives made an assessment of need in 78 cases, and in hospital 3 the midwives made an assessment in 48 cases.

It is notable that hospital 1, which had the highest percentage of mothers visited in the antenatal period, also had the highest percentage of mothers in social classes 1 and 2.

In hospitals 1 and 3 it was said that mothers could exercise some degree of choice about the length of time they stayed in hospital after the birth of their babies, but in hospital 2 a more rigid policy was pursued with all primigravid mothers being expected to stay in hospital or a GP maternity unit for a minimum of seven days. When the mothers were asked 'Did you have a choice in the length of stay in the postnatal ward?', 129 (47 per cent of the total sample) said that they thought they had a choice;

the highest percentage of these mothers was in hospital 1 where they had been visited by a community midwife. This is probably due to the facility provided for the mother to discuss her needs fully with community midwife and then to review her decision near to the expected date of delivery. The arrangements for transfer home were more flexible in hospital 3 than in the other two hospitals.

One mother's comments upon the difficulty of reaching and being held to a decision taken early in pregnancy reflects the frustration which can occur.

> I feel it is very hard to know when you are only three or four months pregnant how long you will need to stay in hospital. I had ten days in hospital with my first baby - bearing this in mind I asked for seven days. But this time I could cope much better and felt well enough to go home after three or four days. I soon found out, however, that seven day bookings remain seven day bookings!

Another difficulty created by the system of deciding the time of transfer early in pregnancy is that any change which requires the mother to stay longer than was planned causes considerable distress. This tended to happen most frequently when the planned discharge was delayed because the baby had developed jaundice.

However, in spite of these observations most mothers felt that the length of time spent in hospital had been satisfactory. When the mothers were asked to comment six weeks after the birth on the length of time that they had stayed in hospital, 219 (78.5 per cent) felt that their stay had been about the right length of time, 37 (13.3 per cent) said it had been too long and 20 (7.2 per cent) said it had been too short.

Arrangements for transfer home and community care

Of the mothers, 233 (83.5 per cent of the total sample) were transferred home before the baby was a week old, and of these 167 (59.9 per cent) were transferred on or before the third day after the baby's birth. Of the 167 mothers, 49 (17.6 per cent of the total sample) were transferred to a GP maternity unit before going to the care of the community midwife. The midwives often expressed frustration at the rapid turnover of mothers and babies passing through the postnatal wards, and said that this prevented them from giving individualized care to their clients.

It was not uncommon for the midwife who was arranging for a mother to go home to have had little or no direct contact with her in the preceding days. In all three hospitals a system operated whereby the midwife in charge of the ward automatically took responsibility for arranging for mothers to go home, and this routine pattern continued even when the midwife in charge had been off duty for the period immediately before the day of discharge. These midwives then relied upon the written notes, and when possible they consulted with their colleagues who had come direct knowledge of each particular mother. The transfer system, however, tended to be very routine in its approach, relying mainly on the arrangements made with the community midwife during the antenatal period. These arrangements were usually implemented without question unless the mother or baby were considered to be 'having problems'. 'Problems' were usually defined as difficulty in feeding, or the baby having some degree of jaundice. Very rarely was the mother's level of confidence taken into consideration.

When the mother was transferred to the care of the community midwife very little information about her progress in the feeding or care of her baby was included on the routine information which was sent to the midwife concerned. Occasionally the hospital midwife would discuss a mother with the community midwife via the telephone, but this was usually done in cases where some problem had occurred to do with the time of transfer home or the amount of help the mother could expect on her return home. All the hospitals had a prepared form on which information was sent to the community midwife concerning the date of birth of the baby, details of the labour and delivery, blood samples taken from the mother and baby, and the type of feeding and time of transfer home. The standardized nature of these forms allowed very little opportunity to give further information.

The most usual person to care for the mother on her return home was her husband (40 per cent of the sample), followed by her mother or mother-in-law (31 per cent). A number of mothers (17.6 per cent) were looked after by both husband and mother or mother-in-law, and the rest were cared for by other relatives or friends (9.2 per cent) or by no one (2.2 per cent).

Midwives perception of the mothers during postnatal care at home

The community midwives visited 44 per cent of the mothers on the same day that they were discharged from hospital, and a further 52.3 per cent of the mothers were visited on the morning of the day after discharge from the hospital.

They described 54 mothers as showing signs of emotional distress after their transfer home from hospital, and of these 17 were said to have 'third day blues' while 37 had distress due to other circumstances such as physical discomfort or lack of sleep. The community midwives noted 49 mothers as being tearful, 74 as not having enough sleep, 33 as showing undue fatigue, 27 as having signs of irritability and 17 as having poor appetite. They also noted that lack of sleep and undue fatigue affected mothers in the 30+ age group more than any other, but apart from that distinction there were no differences in the age, parity or social class of mothers showing signs of emotional distress.

At the time of discharge from the community midwifery service the midwives considered that family support for the mother had been 'very good' for 67.9 per cent of the mothers, and 'good' for a further 26.6 per cent.

At the time of transfer from hospital 161 babies (59 per cent) were totally breastfed, 93 (34.0 per cent) totally bottlefed and 19 (7.0 per cent) were being breastfed and receiving complementary bottlefeeds as well. (No information available for six babies.) The community midwives reported that 31 mothers had changed their method of feeding after they arrived home. Unfortunately the community midwife report was not received for 44 mothers, and this prevents a detailed analysis of changes for individual mothers. However, at the time when the mothers were discharged from the care of the community midwife 113 (48.0 per cent of those reported) were feeding their babies by breast only, 108 (46.0 per cent) were bottlefeeding, and 14 mothers (six per cent) were still giving breastfeeds topped up with bottlefeeds.

Continuity of care from one or two midwives was more usual in the community. The midwives reported that 59.9 per cent of the mothers had been attended throughout their period of domiciliary care by only two different midwives, and 29 per cent of the mothers were attended by three different midwives. Seventy-six per cent of the mothers were visited by their health visitor during the time when the midwife was giving daily postnatal care.

The trend for midwives to visit mothers at home for longer than the statutory minimum of ten days is shown in the report of the length of domiciliary care (Table 5.7). Only seven mothers (three per cent) were discharged on the tenth day after the baby's birth, and 69 (29.6 per cent) were discharged between 11 and 20 days after the birth. Of the mothers, 131 (56.2 per cent) were discharged between the 21st and 28th day after the birth. The remaining 26 mothers (11.2 per cent) for whom data was obtained were discharged by the 35th day after the birth.

Table 5.7:Differences between hospitals in the length of community care

Time of discharge from care of community midwife	Hospital 1		Hospital 2		Hospital 3		Total Sample	
	n	%	n	%	n	%	n	%
On 10th day	2	1.9	2	2.3	3	7.3	7	3.0
11-20 days	2	1.9	42	48.3	25	61.0	69	29.6
21-28 days	85	81.0	37	42.5	9	22.0	131	56.2
29-35 days	16	15.2	6	6.8	4	9.8	26	11.1
Total[a]	105	100.0	86	100.0	41	100.0	233	100.0

$$x^2 = 82.78174, \text{ 8d.f.;}\ P = 0.0001$$

[a]   Missing cases = 46

The pattern of postnatal care reported in this chapter is typical of that provided by the maternity services of the National Health Service at the present time. The majority of mothers are transferred to the care of the community midwife two or three days after the birth of the baby. The bulk of postnatal care therefore takes place in the community. Although the pattern of early transfer home has been typical of maternity care for a number of years, the continuation of community care beyond the tenth postnatal day was in 1980 a comparatively recent development.

CHAPTER 6

Analysing the Results: Factors Associated with Emotional Well-being and Satisfaction with Motherhood

The purpose of the study was to examine the effects which the postnatal support given to mothers by midwives might have upon maternal emotional well-being, and to consider the role played by midwives in the light of factors which had been found significant in other studies of postnatal emotional status and satisfaction. All the data therefore were analysed to discover the existence and strength of links between any of the maternal or family factors, the events of the birth and the postnatal period, and the mothers emotional well-being and satisfaction with motherhood measured 6-8 weeks after the birth.

Of the total sample of 279 mothers; 30 (10.7 per cent) were very happy and well-adjusted, 195 (69.9 per cent) were coping well, and 54 women (19.4 per cent) were classified as being emotionally distressed or on the verge of postnatal depression. This proportion of emotionally distressed mothers is consistent with that found in many other studies (Pitt, 1968; Paykel, 1980; Kumar and Robson, 1984).

The significance of these results and the main factors associated with them is discussed in the following chapter. A summary of the main findings is listed below.

Factors/ events linked to emotional well-being

Antecedent factors
- Personality - degree of trait anxiety measured by the EPI
- Presence of life-stress events

Other stresses/factors
- Feelings at time of birth
- Self-image in feeding baby while in hospital care
- Conflicting advice/ rest in hospital

Self-confidence on return home from hospital
- Family support at home
- Degree of satisfaction with motherhood six weeks after birth

Factors/events not linked to emotional well-being
- Age, parity or social class of mother
- Separation from own mother before 11 years of age
- Planning/not planning pregnancy
- Events of labour or delivery
- Choice of feeding pattern
- Pattern of postnatal care; length of stay in hospital, length of visiting by community midwife

Defining emotional well-being
The measures of emotional well-being, satisfaction with motherhood and perception of postnatal care were obtained from the mothers' answers to the various statements which made up the postnatal questionnaire.

The factor analysis of the questionnaire, which is described in Chapter 4, indicated that the answers to 23 statements clustered together to form five emotional well-being factors. These factors were: depression, including loss of libido; coping ability; anxiety sleep disturbance associated with anxiety; and self-confidence. The scores given on each of these factors were added together to form the emotional well-being (EWB) score. (For details of the scoring system see page 44.

The results were as listed below.

- The range of possible EWB scores was from 23 to 115.
- The range of actual EWB scores was from 46 to 108.
- The mean average EWB score was 78.179.
- The standard deviation was 7.516.

Although wherever possible the whole range of EWB scores was used in the analysis of the results, it was necessary in defining low, moderate and high emotional well-being, both to assist certain methods of analysis and to compare the women classed as having low emotional well-being with those described by earlier research. In order to do so the following methods were used.

Women who had a total EWB score of 68 of less, which represents a mean average score of 2.95 or less per statement, were defined as the low emotional well-being group and considered to be emotionally distressed. There were 54 women in this group and they formed 19.4 per cent of the total sample.

Women with low emotional well-being
The scores of the women who formed the low emotional well-being group revealed that they had symptoms similar to those of the depressed group described by Pitt

(1968). They exhibited depression, anxiety and guilt (especially about the baby), sleep disturbance, tiredness, and lack of confidence in their ability to cope with the needs of the baby. All the babies were thriving at the time when the mothers completed the emotional well-being questionnaire.

There were other similarities between the emotionally distressed group in this study and those described by Pitt. He noted that the depressed women in his study had felt physically unwell in the early post-partum period, and that these feelings were quite distinct from those of the 'third day blues'. Their depression, which began in the hospital and grew worse when they first returned home with the baby, was experienced chiefly as tearfulness, feelings of inadequacy and inability to cope.

A similar picture was seen when a mother's score on the postnatal care questionnaire was examined in relation to her EWB score. Women whose scores for postnatal care in hospital indicated that they had not felt fit and well during their stay in hospital had significantly lower EWB scores, and a further significant relationship was found between their scores for self-confidence when they returned home with the baby and their EWB scores.

One of the problems of assessing emotional well-being is the different cut-off points used to define distress or depression. In studies undertaken by psychiatrists the scales used have clear diagnostic criteria, and many women who are severely distressed might not actually fulfil these criteria. This "tip of the iceberg" can be seen in Pitt's study (1968). He considered that 10.8 per cent of his sample of 305 women were depressed, but noted that a further ten per cent were considerably distressed, and he describes them as "doubtfully depressed". It is likely that many of the mothers classed as emotionally distressed in this study would have come into Pitt's category of "doubtfully depressed", although some were considered to be depressed on the basis of their responses on the Beck Depression Inventory statements. Whatever the criteria, these women were unhappy and miserable at a time when most were coping well and some were extremely happy and well-adjusted.

The similarities which exist between Pitt's description of mothers suffering from 'atypical depression', the criteria of depression included in the Beck Depression Inventory and the scoring patterns of the emotionally distressed group in this study suggest that the emotional well-being questionnaire was an effective tool in differentiating between the different levels of emotional well-being expressed by the 279 women who formed the total sample.

It must be recognized that the mother's feelings at the time of completing the questionnaire would have had a marked effect upon her responses, and care must be taken to distinguish between results which may be considered to be a further reflection of her emotional state at that time and those which indicate other factors and events which contributed to emotional outcome. The analysis of the results was therefore designed to assess the relationship which a variety of factors and events had with the different levels of maternal emotional well-being.

Analysing the results

In the analysis of the results three main approaches were used. In some situations the whole range of EWB scores were analysed against the range of other scores, for example the Eysenck Personality Inventory (EPI) or the other factor scores such as rest in hospital, or satisfaction with motherhood. In these situations rank correlation methods were used. The other methods used were chi-square analysis, where the EWB scores were grouped as high, medium or low and analysed against events such as type of labour or delivery. The most frequently usedmethods were the Mann-Whitney U test (M-W) and the Kruskall-Wallis one-way analysis of variance by ranks (K-W). Both of these rank observations in order from the lowest to the highest and then determine whether the rank order of two or more different groups is so different that the groups are not likely to come from the same population. For example, the Mann-Whitney test was used to analyse the effect of parity on the rank order of the mother's score on the pain in labour scale. Primigravidae were put in group 1, multiparae in group 2. The results showed that most of the group 1 scores fell in the lower ranks while most of the group 2 scores were in the middle and higher ranks. The probability that the scores came from the same population was assessed as less than 0.01, indicating that the difference between the two groups was statistically significant and not due to underlying random error. The use of statistical methods reduces the danger that the researcher's own opinions on, for example, parity and the mechanisms of labour, would result in a biased judgement of the significance of the results based upon subjective feelings rather than well-grounded evidence.

Overview of the results

Three main parameters were identified, each of which contributed to the mother's emotional well-being but which arose from differing circumstances. For the sake of clarity it is necessary to discuss these parameters separately, but it must be remembered that they were part of a complex and dynamic interactive process in which some factors were seen to increase emotional conflict while others reduced it.

The three main parameters are listed below.

1. **Anxiety and its effects.**
   There was a close relationship between anxiety and emotional outcome which also affected maternal perception of self-confidence and support, but not satisfaction with motherhood.

2. **Stress related to life-crises and postnatal care.**
   The coping process was affected by additional stress arising from certain life-crisis events and particular aspects of postnatal care.

3. **Satisfaction with motherhood.**
   A relationship between emotional well-being and satisfaction with motherhood indicated that maternal satisfaction may increase emotional well-being but is itself affected by factors in the mother and in the management of her care.

These will all be discussed in detail below.

Factors which were not related to emotional outcome

The analysis also revealed that a number of major variables were not related to emotional well-being.

- The personality trait of extroversion/introversion measured by the Eysenck Personality Inventory approximately four weeks before the birth of the baby.
- Maternal separation from her own mother before the age of 11 years.
- The age and parity of the mother.
- The type of labour and delivery experienced by the mother.
- The time the mother spent in hospital.
- The time for which the mother was visited by the community midwife.

The Eysenck Personality Inventory (EPI) is a trait test of extroversion/ introversion and neuroticism/anxiety. (Eysenck and Eysenck, 1968; Eysenck, Soueif and White, 1969). The client's response to a series of questions produces two scores: the 'E' score, which gives a measure of extroversion/introversion; and the 'N' score, which is a measure of neuroticism/anxiety.

Extroversion/introversion

In the initial analysis of the results of individual hospitals, no significant relationship was found between the mothers' score on the extroversion/introversion scale on the EPI and her eventual EWB scores.

There were no significant differences in the distribution of either the extroversion/ introversion scores or the anxiety/neuroticism scores of the mothers cared for by the three different hospitals, and the extroversion/introversion scores were eliminated from further analysis.

Separation

Although Frommer and O'Shea (1973) found that women separated from their mothers before the age of 11 years were more likely to have difficulty in adjusting to motherhood, no significant differences were found between the EWB scores of the 33 women in this study who reported such separation and the remainder of the sample who did not (M-W test; P = 0.4664). There was, however, a marked difference between the EPI anxiety/neuroticism (EPI(N)) scores of the separated women and the non-separated women (M-W test; P = 0.0002). This suggests that the separation had an effect upon the developing personality of the women concerned, adding weight to Brown and Harris's (1978) conclusion that separation is a predisposing factor in the incidence of depression among vulnerable women (see Table 6.1.)

Age and parity

There were no significant differences in the mothers' EWB scores as a result of age or parity (see Table 6.2).

Table 6.1:EPI(N) scores and EWB scores classified by separation/non-separation from own mother before the age of 11 years (Mann-Whitney U test corrected for ties)

	EPI(N)		EWB	
	n	Mean rank score	n	Mean rank score
Separated from own mother	32	180.6	33	128.5
Not separated from own mother	233	126.4	242	139.3
	z = 3.7714; P = 0.0002		z = -0.7283; P = 0.4664	

Table 6.2:EPI(N) scores and EWB scores classified by age, parity, type of labour and delivery

Variable	EPI(N)		EWB	
	n	Mean rank score	n	Mean rank score
Age of mother				
17-20 years	30	146.7	31	146.4
21-30 years	155	140.4	164	135.3
31-39 years	83	119.1	84	146.8
	K-W test: x^2 = 4.9598; P = 0.0838		x^2 = 1.3637; P = 0.5057	
Parity				
Primigravidae	92	134.6	98	142.6
Multiparae	175	133.7	179	137.0
	M-W test: z = 0.0995; P = 0.9208		z = -0.5485; P = 0.5833	
Type of labour				
Spontaneous	116	131.8	123	133.0
Induced	94	130.6	97	150.4
Actively managed	57	144.1	58	135.0
	K-W test: x^2 = 1.2468; P = 0.5361		x^2 = 2.7696; P = 0.2504	
Type of delivery				
Normal	188	136.4	195	142.8
Forceps	47	132.3	50	132.2
Breech	4	99.5	4	34.0
Caesarian	28	125.9	29	144.3
	K-W test: x^2 = 1.3156; P = 0.7254		x^2 = 7.7362; P = 0.0518	

Labour and delivery

Women who had an induced labour scored higher mean average EWB scores than those who had either normal or actively managed labour, but the difference was not statistically significant (K-W test; P = 0.2504). (Women who had a caesarean section were included in the actively managed group.)

There were virtually no differences in the EWB scores of women who had a normal delivery, a forceps delivery or a caesarean section, but the four women who had a breech delivery scored very low EWB scores. A weak statistically significant difference was noted between the scores of the women in the breech group and those who had other forms of delivery, but this is distorted by the extremely small number concerned. It is concluded, therefore, that there was no significant relationship between emotional well-being and the form of labour or delivery the mother experienced. (Details of these results can be seen in Table 6.2.)

Factors which were significantly related to postnatal emotional well-being

The three main factors which were found to be significantly related to postnatal emotional well-being were anxiety as an antecedent factor, stress associated with concurrent life-crisis events, and stress associated with certain aspects of postnatal care.

Anxiety and its wide-ranging effects

Although the personality trait of extroversion/introversion was not significantly associated with postnatal emotional well-being, that of trait anxiety was highly significant. Anxiety affected the mother's perception of her care in hospital and of the support she received from her family when she returned home. High levels of trait anxiety were associated with lower social class and bottlefeeding.

Anxiety as an antecedent factor

A strong relationship was found between a mother's EWB score recorded six weeks after the baby was born and her level of anxiety measured by the anxiety/neuroticism (N) scale on the EPI approximately four weeks before the baby was born (K-W test; P = 0.0001).

As can be seen from Table 6.3, mothers in the low emotional well-being group had much higher EPI(N) scores than the rest of the sample. This link between anxiety/neuroticism and emotional well-being provided further confirmation of the similarity between the results of this study and those of Pitt's study (1968). He found a significant relationship between postnatal depression and high anxiety/neuroticism scores measured on the Maudsley Medical Inventory (Eysenck, 1959), which was the forerunner of the EPI (Eysenck and Eysenck, 1986).

Table 6.3:EPI(N) scores compared with post-natal EWB scores (Kruskall-Wallis one-way analysis of variance)

EWB	n	EPI(N) Mean rank score
Low scores	54	186.4
Moderate scores	187	125.7
High scores	27	91.6
	K-W test: x^2 = 35.0252; P = 0.0001	

This result amply illustrates Lazarus's contention that anxiety is a powerful force in the coping process and that it may be present both as an antecedent factor in the form of a personality trait and as a contributory factor in the form of state anxiety aroused in response to stress (Lazarus, 1966, 1969).

Kumar and Robson (1978, 1984) used the EPI to assess the relationship between personality and postnatal depression in a sample of 119 primigravidae. In their study the EPI was completed during the first trimester of pregnancy and the assessment of postnatal depression was undertaken three months post-delivery. Kumar and Robson did not find a significant relationship between high EPI(N) scores and postnatal depression. Although the difference in the timing of the two measures makes direct comparison difficult, their results suggest that any relationship between trait anxiety and emotional distress reduces with the passage of time. If this is so, then it is an indication that anxious women need a longer time than less anxious women to adapt to motherhood.

People with high trait anxiety as measured by the EPI are not highly neurotic, but can be described as timid, fearful, very sensitive to criticism and anxious to please. Women generally score higher than men, and working class people score higher than any other social class (Eysenck and Eysenck, 1968; Eysenck et a*l*, 1969).

Anxiety and social class
The link between anxiety and social class is another indication of the complexity of the situation surrounding vulnerability to depression (Brown and Harris, 1978) and it emerged in he results of this study. The mothers in social classes 3 manual (m), 4 and 5 had higher EPI(N) scores than those in social classes 1, 2 and 3 non-manual (n/m) (M-W test; P = 0.003). The mothers in social classes 3m, 4 and 5 also had lower EWB scores than the women in social classes 1, 2 and 3 n/m (M-W test; P = 0.0038). However, the degree of statistical significance of the correlation between social class and anxiety is higher than that between social class and emotional well-being, and this suggests that the link between social class and emotional well-being can be attributed to the underlying personality factor. The details of the relationship between social class, personality, emotional well-being and choice of infant feeding method are given in Table 6.4.

Table 6.4:EPI(N) scores and EWB scores classified by social class and choice of infant feeding method

Variable	EPI(N)		EWB	
	n	Mean rank score	n	Mean rank score
Social class [a]				
1 and 2	83	107.3	85	141.4
3n/m	38	118.1	39	162.7
3m	61	137.9	68	123.1
4	51	153.0	51	120.2
5	23	142.8	23	115.2
	K-W test: $x^2 = 15.0342$; $P = 0.0046$		$x^2 = 10.6218$; $P = 0.0312$	
Choice of feeding method				
Breast	156	119.0	161	146.2
Bottle	106	149.9	112	123.8
	M-W test: $z = -3.2431$; $P = 0.0012$		$z = 2.3068$; $P = 0.0211$	

[a] Eleven unclassified mothers not included

Anxiety and choice of feeding method

The close relationship between anxiety and social class described above was found to be a factor in the difference between the EWB scores of the mothers who breastfed their babies and those who bottlefed (see Table 6.4). Working class mothers are known to choose bottlefeeding more often than breastfeeding (Bacon and Wylie, 1976; Houston, 1981; Thomson, 1989). In the present study 51.4 per cent of the mothers in social classes 3m, 4 and 5 chose to bottlefeed their babies compared with 12.5 per cent of the mothers in social classes 1, 2 and 3 n/m. Mothers of all social classes who bottlefed their babies had higher EPI(N) scores before the baby was born (M-W test; p = 0.0012) and lower EWB scores six weeks after delivery than the breastfeeding mothers (M-W test; P = 0.0211). Once again the degree of difference between anxiety and choice of feeding method is greater than between emotional well-being and feeding method, indicating that the link between anxiety and social class is also a factor in the choice of infant feeding method. If this is so then it brings a new dimension into the approach which professional staff should have towards encouraging women to breastfeed their babies. The anxious woman may choose to bottlefeed in order to avoid the effect which she perceives the difficulty of breastfeeding may have upon her fragile coping resources. Any overt disapproval of her choice will cause guilt and distress and is likely to undermine her confidence.

Anxiety and adjustment to motherhood

Another set of interactive relationships was found between a mother's antenatal EPI(N) scores, her feelings of physical and emotional well-being in the postnatal ward, her self-confidence and perception of support when she returned home and her emotional well-being six weeks after delivery. The physical well-being factor score indicated whether or not the mother had felt fit and well during the time she spent in the postnatal ward. The ward-atmosphere factor score indicated her feelings about being in the hospital; whether she felt relaxed and at home, freely able to ask questions and obtain help, or whether she felt homesick and lonely, and afraid to ask questions.

The mothers who gave low scores on these factors had significantly higher EPI(N) scores than the rest of the sample, and they also had lower EWB scores (see Table 6.5). The anxious women found it less easy to relax and feel at home in the ward, and their anxiety was manifested in physical as well as emotional symptoms. There is no evidence to suggest that the anxious mothers received poorer care than the rest of the mothers in the same ward, but their natural anxiety made it more difficult for them to cope with the strange environment.

Table 6.5:EPI(N) scores and EWB scores compared with scores for postnatal ward atmosphere and physical well-being

Variable	EPI(N)		EWB	
	n	Mean rank score	n	Mean rank score
Ward atmosphere	78	153.4	77	102.9
Moderate scores	115	130.6	125	146.4
High scores	75	120.8	77	155.5
	K-W test: $x^2 = 7.3102$; $P = 0.0259$		$x^2 = 15.7959$; $P = 0.0004$	
Physical well-being				
Low scores	44	156.5	46	95.7
Moderate/high scores	224	130.2	233	148.8
	M-W test: $z = 2.0624$; $P = 0.0392$		$z = -4.0802$; $P = 0.0001$	

The study of medical patients provides further evidence of the difficulty which people with high trait anxiety have in adjusting to hospital. In a study by Wilson-Barnett and Carrigy (1978) the trait anxiety levels of non-urgent medical patients admitted to one ward were assessed on the (N) scale of the EPI on the day of their admission to hospital. The patients' state anxiety was then assessed daily by the Lishman Mood Adjective List (Lishman, 1972) for as long as they remained in the hospital. The patients who had high EPI(N) scores on the day of admission manifested much higher levels of state anxiety than the other patients in the same ward, and their anxiety remained high for at least five days after admission.

Anxious people find it difficult to relax, to take in information and to learn new skills. It is unrealistic, therefore, to expect anxious mothers to learn how to care for their babies and to cope with carrying out that care at the same pace as less anxious mothers. They will need more time to become confident and may need to have the same information imparted on a number of occasions before they make full use of it. Anxious people become more anxious when they feel that they are not conforming with others' expectations of them.

The interactive relationship between trait anxiety and emotional well-being is seen again in the mother's scores for self-confidence and perception of family support when she returned home with the baby (see Table 6.6). The mothers who scored low on these factors had higher EPI(N) scores and lower EWB scores than the other mothers.

Table 6.6:EPI(N) scores and EWB scores compared with scores for self-confidence and family support at home (Mann-Whitney U test corrected for ties)

		EPI(N)	EWB
Variable	*n*	Mean rank score	Mean rank score
Self-confidence at home			
Low scores	28	163.4	45.3
Moderate/high scores	240	131.1	146.5
M-W test: $z = 2.0807$; $P = 0.0369$		$z = -5.1490$; $P = 0.0001$	
Family support at home			
Low scores	76	156.9	90.3
Moderate/high scores	188	122.6	155.4
M-W test: $z = 3.3079$; $P = 0.0009$		$z = -5.7278$; $P = 0.0001$	

The reports from the community midwives support the mother's retrospective rating of her confidence when she returned home with the baby. They recorded that 54 mothers had shown signs of emotional distress within a few days of their return from the hospital. Six weeks later these mothers rated their self-confidence in the early days at home as poor, and their scores were significantly lower than those of the rest of the sample (M-W test; $P = 0.0060$).

Mothers who rated the quality of their support from their families as low, also had higher EPI(N) scores (M-W test; $P = 0.0009$) and lower EWB scores than any other group (M-W test; $P = 0.0001$) (see Table 6.7). This time the community midwives' assessment of the quality of the support the mother received from her family did not coincide with that of the mother, suggesting that it is not the amount of support which matters to the mother but the quality of that support in relation to her emotional needs and confidence.

There is no doubt that personality was a powerful influence upon the way women coped with the demands of motherhood, and that anxious women were more vulnerable to emotional distress.

Pitt's study (1968) found a similar pattern of physical and emotional distress, lack of confidence and dissatisfaction with family support among his depressed mothers. It is difficult to determine to what extent the low scores for physical and emotional well-being in the ward and lack of confidence and family support at home were due to the underlying effect of high anxiety and to what extent these feelings were signs of developing postnatal distress.

Table 6.7: Mothers' scores for self-confidence , family support, emotional well-being and satisfaction with motherhood classified by midwives' observations of maternal emotional distress during the first week at home (Mann-Whitney U test corrected for ties)

Factors	Midwives' observations	
	Emotional distress seen (mean rank scores; $n = 54$)	Emotional distress not seen (mean rank scores; $n = 183$)
Self-confidence	97.1	125.5
	$z = -2.7504$; $P = 0.0060$	
Family support	108.9	122.0
	$z = 1.2612$; $P = 0.2072$	
Emotional well-being	104.0	123.4
	$z = -1.8294$; $P = 0.0673$	
Satisfaction with motherhood	116.2	119.8
	$z = -0.3455$; $P = 0.7297$	

The high degree of significance between the scores for the postnatal care factors and the EWB scores suggests that many of the mothers who felt unwell and unhappy in hospital and who lacked confidence at home were showing early signs of the emotional distress which was still present six weeks later.

Many mothers experience some degree of emotional disturbance in the early postnatal period, but this usually passes as confidence grows. For a number of vulnerable women, however, this distress did not pass away but signalled a spiralling situation of anxiety, lack of confidence and emotional distress.

Stressful life-events

The main focus of this study is the major life-event of pregnancy, childbirth and the mothering of a new infant. It would be foolish, however, to assume that this was the only major life-event being experienced by the mothers and their families, and many of the mothers in the sample reported other life-crises which had occurred during the year preceding the birth of the baby. These included the death or serious illness of a close family member, marriage or the separation of couples, changes in the mother's or her partner's employment, and either moving house or having major alterations done to the house. In addition, the mothers volunteered information about other stressful events. These fell into two main categories: marital and family conflict, and difficulty in adjusting to the loss of an interesting career.

Altogether 456 life-events were reported by the 279 mothers in the study. For many of them, therefore, the birth of a baby was one more stressful event to cope with in an existing situation of adjustment and stress.

The relationship between life-events and emotional well being is shown in Table 6.8. It can be seen that there were no significant differences in the EWB scores of women who reported the death or illness of a family member, marriage or separation, or changes in the partner's employment compared with women who did not suffer these stresses. But women who reported marital tension or a disturbance to the home, i.e. moving house or having major alterations done, scored significantly lower levels of emotional well-being. The degree of significance between the scores of the mothers who moved house and those who did not is not high; this life-event is included because it affected 112 mothers (40 per cent of the sample) and because an association between moving house and severe postnatal depression has been observed in clinical practice (Oates, personal communication, 1984) and in the study by Paykel *et al* (1980).

Table 6.8:EWB scores classified by life-crisis events (Mann-Whitney U test corrected for ties)

		EWB	
Life-crisis	*n*	Mean rank score	
Death of close family			
Yes	61	123.6	
No	211	132.4	
		$z = 1.6177$; $P = 0.1057$	
Marriage changes			
Yes	37	123.6	
No	233	137.4	
		$z = 0.9988$; $P = 0.3179$	
Illness in close family			
Yes	66	128.9	
No	205	138.3	
		$z = -0.8464$; $P = 0.3973$	
Moved house			
Yes	112	125.4	
No	160	144.3	
		$z = -1.9461$; $P = 0.0516$	
Changes in husband's work			
Yes	90	120.9	
No	173	137.9	
		$z = -1.7009$; $P = 0.0890$	
Marital tension/giving up work			
Yes	90	115.1	
No	181	146.4	
		$z = -3.0953$; $P = 0.0020$	

Marital conflict

A relationship between marital conflict and depression in women has been demonstrated in other studies of postnatal difficulties (Tod, 1964; Nuckalls et al, 1972; Kumar and Robson, 1978, 1984; Paykel et al, 1980; O'Hara et al, 1983, 1984; Oakley, 1980), and in a study of the role of social factors in the incidence of depression in women (Brown and Harris 1978, Stein et al, 1989). It has its basis in the lack of a warm confiding relationship that leads to feelings of vulnerability and lack of self-esteem or self-worth which makes support ineffective if not impossible. If unrelieved, these feelings lead to a degree of apathy and fear of further failure which renders women helpless and unable to change their situation.

Adjusting to giving up work

The other main area of conflict was reported by women who said they were finding difficulty in adjusting to being at home all day after giving up an interesting job and working environment. Several mothers commented about their feelings on this matter when they completed the postnatal questionnaire six weeks after the post-delivery interview. One commented that:

> In spite of having a devoted and helpful husband I find loving our baby difficult still, and feel trapped when my husband goes out to work. I never realized how much freedom I'd lose having a baby.

Another mother, who had just left her post as a social worker said:

> Being a mother is satisfying and totally exhausting and downgraded and not appreciated by our society!

Oakley (1980) argues that the primary loss in becoming a mother is loss of identity. Giving up an interesting and rewarding job is a loss of the mother's identity as a capable and valued member of the working population. Her competence in her chosen career is replaced at least initially by her 'apprenticeship' at the new job of motherhood. This loss of identity is made worse by a society which does not value the contribution made by all parents in the nurture of its future citizens. Leaving work also entails leaving the peer support of colleagues at a time when the opportunity to make new friends is restricted by the needs of a new baby.

Moving house

Women who moved house also suffered loss of identity and loss of peer support. Paykel et al (1980) also found moving house to be a significant factor in postnatal depression but considered that its main impact was secondary to other stress such as marital tension. However, when we consider how big the impact of moving house generally is for a woman, perhaps it should be given a higher priority. Often the house is the woman's particular territory, the place where her personality and values have most expression and the place where she has primary control over the lifestyle of her family. The term 'housewife' is indicative of the way society identifies the role of women with the house in which they live, in a way which would be unthinkable if applied to men. Moving house disrupts the lifestyle and considerable effort and organization is required before new patterns of living can be established. It also separates the mother from the support of family and friends in the area left behind, and this loss of support increases the likelihood that the mother's own needs will be submerged beneath those of her baby and the rest of her family to a considerable degree.

The life-events described above all increased the amounts of stress with which the affected mothers were coping, by reducing the amount and quality of family or peer support which was available to them, and thus making them increasingly vulnerable to emotional distress.

Reviewing the hypotheses

The research design was based upon two hypotheses (see Chapter 4). The first hypothesis stated that:

> the emotional response of women to the changes which follow the birth of a child will be affected by their personality and by the quality of the support they receive from family and social support systems.

The results analysis discussed in this chapter upholds this hypothesis and illustrates the way in which factors in the mother and in her personal family situation affected her adjustment to motherhood.

The second hypothesis stated that:

> the way in which care is provided by midwives during the postnatal period will influence the emotional response of women to the changes which follow the birth of a child.

The study also identified factors which upheld the second hypothesis and which were related to the mother's feelings about her baby, her competence as a mother, and to the way in which care was given by midwives working in hospital.

Postnatal care factors which contributed to emotional well-being

The analysis of the results revealed two other factors which contributed to the vulnerability of mothers to depression. These were both identified from the mothers' assessments of the postnatal care received in hospital, and were maternal self-image in feeding and the amount of rest received during the stay in hospital.

A mother's score for these factors was significantly related to her EWB score but not to her personality trait nor to the degree of satisfaction she had with motherhood. This suggests that they were evidence of extra stress (lack of sleep) and/or early signs of emerging distress (self-image in feeding). In either case, the evidence suggests that they could be reduced or prevented by more sympathetic postnatal care. Details are given in table 6.9.

Table 6.9:EPI(N) scores, satisfaction with motherhood and EWB scores compared with scores for self-image in feeding and rest in hospital (Mann-Whitney U test corrected for ties)

	EPI(N)		Satisfaction with motherhood		EWB	
	n	Mean rank score	n	Mean rank score	n	Mean rank score
Self-image in feeding						
Low scores	62	132.1	61	132.1	63	93.0
Moderate/high scores	206	130.4	215	136.5	213	147.0
	$z = 1.5981$; $P = 0.1100$		$z = 1.3701$; $P = 0.1707$		$z = -3.7501$; $P = 0.0002$	
Rest in hospital						
Low scores	114	136.5	121	129.4	118	125.7
Moderate/high scores	154	133.0	156	143.5	161	150.5
	$z = 0.3619$; $P = 0.7174$		$z = -1.5572$; $P = 0.1192$		$z = -2.5297$; $P = 0.0114$	

Self-image in feeding - midwives observations

The self-image in feeding factor was quite separate from the feeding support factor, which reflected the mother's perception of the quality of support she received from midwives and other members of the nursing staff when feeding her baby. Instead it reflected her feelings and judgement of her own competence in feeding her baby, compared with that of other mothers in the same ward.

Depressed people are very self-critical and it might be considered that this was the reason for the strong relationship between low self-image in feeding scores and low EWB scores. There was, however, considerable evidence that this was not so, but that the self-image score reflected the mother's feelings during the early postnatal period rather than her feelings at the time when she completed the questionnaire.

The self-image in feeding scores were related to the mothers' level of experience of feeding a baby and to real difficulties which she encountered in feeding her baby and which were observed by the hospital midwives. The scores of primigravidae early in the postnatal period were accordingly significantly lower than those of the multiparous women, reflecting their lack of experience and competence in feeding a baby. Six weeks later, though, the EWB scores of primigravidae were not significantly different from those of the multiparae - in fact they were slightly higher.

The hospital midwives' reports confirmed the reality of the mother's feelings as revealed in her self- image in feeding score. During the interview held with a hospital midwife on the day each mother was discharged from hospital, the midwives had identified 54 mothers who had been 'unduly' distressed about feeding their babies and who had needed more than the 'normal' amount of help. Six weeks later these mothers scored significantly lower scores on the self-image in feeding factor than the rest of the sample.

Of these 54 mothers, 30 were breastfeeding and 24 were bottlefeeding their infants. The distressed mothers did not have higher EPI(N) scores, which means that the distress was not the result of high trait anxiety. Neither were the EWB scores markedly different for all of these 54 mothers identified by the midwives, which means that some of them had recovered by six weeks, and others who later rated themselves with low self-image in feeding, were not identified as distressed by the midwives. Details can be seen in Table 6.10. (Information was missing from 10 mothers.)

Table 6.10:EPI(N) scores and scores for self-image in feeding, rest in hospital, emotional well-being and satisfaction with motherhood classified by midwives' observations of maternal distress during feeding in the postnatal ward (Mann-Whitney U test corrected for ties)

	Midwives' observations in postnatal ward	
Factors	Mothers distressed (mean rank scores; n = 54)	Mothers not distressed (mean rank scores; n = 220)
EPI(N)	127.8	133.0
	z = -0.4438; P = 0.6572	
Self-image in feeding	99.5	146.8
	z = -3.9870; P = 0.0001	
Rest in hospital	115.9	142.8
	z = -2.2505; P = 0.0244	
Emotional well-being	135.1	138.1
	z = -0.2483; P = 0.8039	
Satisfaction with motherhood	138.1	137.4
	z = 0.0590; P = 0.9530	

Once again the picture emerges of two groups of mothers within the total group of those who had shown distress about feeding their babies in the early postnatal period. For many of them, initial anxiety was replaced by growing confidence and skill as they and their babies learnt together how to manage feeding. For others, the distress was a manifestation of continuing problems of low self-esteem, and continuing conflict.

A mother's self-image in feeding in hospital was also related to her perception of her baby's progress measured on the Broussard-type scale six weeks later. Mothers were asked to assess whether their baby was better or worse than the 'average' baby in such matters as the number of crying spells, difficulties in feeding, sleeping difficulties and settling down to an expected pattern of behaviour. The concept of 'average' was that of the mother. Table 6.11 shows that 36 mothers thought their babies were doing worse than average on all four counts, 127 thought their baby was doing as well as the average baby and 112 said that their babies were doing better than the average baby, (four mothers did not complete the score). There were statistically significant differences in the self-image in feeding scores of the mothers in the three different groups, those who said their babies were doing worse than the average baby scoring the lowest self-image in feeding scores, and those who said their babies were doing better than average scoring much higher self-image in feeding scores (K-W test; P = 0.0064). The mother's self-image was affected by and affected her perception of her baby.

Table 6.11:EPI(N) scores and scores for self-image in feding, emotional well-being and satisfaction with motherhood compared with the mother's perception of her six-week-old baby (Broussard-type score) (Kruskall-Wallis one-way analysis of variance)

Factors	Mother said baby's progress was:		
	Worse than average (mean rank score; $n = 36$)	Average (mean rank score; $n = 127$)	Better than average (mean rank score; $n = 112$)
EPI(N)	141.7	132.2	128.6
		$x^2 = -0.7913$; $P = 0.6753$	
Self-image in feeding	117.3	127.6	155.1
		$x^2 = 10.0878$; $P = 0.0064$	
Emotional well-being	90.7	140.7	148.9
		$x^2 = 15.1281$; $P = 0.0005$	
Satisfaction with motherhood	10.3	135.8	150.4
		$x^2 = 9.9152$; $P = 0.0070$	

Implications of a low self-image in feeding score

The original study by Broussard and Hartner (1971) indicated that mothers with poor self-image regarded their babies as 'difficult' more often than other mothers. Other studies have noted that low self-esteem in the mother is associated with problems in maternal-child relationships leading to child abuse (Lynch *et al*, 1976; Rosen and Stein, 1980).

The study by Lynch *et al* is particularly interesting because they found the same recognition of potential problems by midwives. The histories of women whose children had been referred to the Register of Children at Risk of Non-accidental Injury were compared with those of controls whose babies had been born in the same hospital and at the same time. It was found that 20 mothers whose children were on the At-Risk Register because of neglect or abuse suffered from a number of interlocking marital and family problems, over which they had little or no control, and that 72 per cent of these mothers had been identified by the hospital midwives who cared for them, as having problems in caring adequately for and mothering their newborn babies. Lynch noted that although these early difficulties in mothering had been seen by the midwives, their potential as an early warning of future problems had not been recognized. The recognition by midwives in this study of problems associated with low maternal self-image in feeding and poor perception of the baby's progress six weeks after leaving the hospital confirm Lynch's contention that the midwives' observations could be used to identify serious potential problems in maternal-child relationships.

This picture of poor self-image which arose from and contributed to difficulties in important personal relationships is reminiscent of Seligman's concept of 'learned helplessness' (Seligman, 1975), in which the victim copes by accepting a painful situation as hopeless and ceases to make any effort to overcome or avoid it. Seligman's studies showed that in the absence of any other help, repeated failures in coping lead to apathy and inaction. He also had some success, however, in reversing this pattern by encouraging his subjects and enabling then to achieve small successes until they began to believe that they could cope with certain situations.

This possibility of effecting change in situations of apathy and failure is most important when we consider the role and practice of professional care-givers, whose purpose is to support and enable those experiencing major change and stress to triumph over it. Positive reinforcement and protection from avoidable stress encourages coping behaviour, but negative reinforcement and exposure to unnecessary stress reduces confidence and frustrates the coping mechanism.
This study revealed areas of negative reinforcement and increased stress when a mother's score for self-image in feeding was compared with her reactions to conflicting advice and insufficient rest in the hospital.

Conflicting advice was one of the major sources of dissatisfaction with postnatal care, especially among primigravidae (Ball, 1984), and acted as a contributory factor in emotional distress. Of the mothers, 109 (39 per cent of the total sample) complained about conflicting advice, and they scored significantly lower self-image in feeding scores than those who did not complain of it (M-W test; P = 0.0024).

For many of the mothers conflicting advice caused considerable distress.

> I was very annoyed that in hospital I didn't get enough help with the feeding. Before the birth everyone encourages breastfeeding, but it seemed that for most of the staff it was too much trouble....much easier to give a bottle. By the time I left hospital I was totally confused and if it wasn't for the help and encouragement of the midwife at home I don't think I would have carried on.

Others found their own way of coping with it:.

> I didn't seem to be able to do anything right, and then one midwife told me to feed the baby whenever he needed it, and another one told me off and said he shouldn't be fed more often than every three hours or else I would get sore nipples. In the end I didn't know what to do, and my mother said take no notice of them. In the end the nasty one went on her weekend off and I could manage all right and the feeding went well after that!

The majority of complaints about conflicting advice concerned the feeding of infants, although they were not solely confined to it.

> All the mothers I spoke to also found the different and sometimes conflicting advice from the midwives confusing and upsetting. I heard two sisters tell one girl in my ward exactly opposite ways of folding cot sheets. This almost reduced her to tears as she was feeling depressed at the time. I felt it was unnecessary to make such an issue of so trivial a matter.

Many of the mothers were annoyed by conflicting advice but able to cope with the frustration it caused them. For others, however, it formed one more straw upon the camel's back contributing to the spiral of lowered self-esteem and emotional distress.

Lack of sleep in hospital

A further stress factor associated with both the mother's self-image in feeding and her emotional well-being six weeks later, was that of insufficient sleep in hospital.

Low scores were recorded by 114 mothers for the rest in hospital factor, and these mothers also had significantly lower self-image in feeding (M-W test; $P = 0.0136$) and EWB scores (M-W test; $P = 0.0114$) than 161 mothers who recorded moderate or high scores for the rest in hospital factor. (No scores were available for four mothers.)

This factor was made up of three statements on the questionnaire about postnatal care in hospital. It was found that mothers in hospital 2 scored much higher levels of satisfaction with the rest factor than mothers in the other two hospitals. When the scores for the three statements which made up the factor were analysed by hospital it was found that there were no significant differences between hospitals for the statements 'It was easy to get enough rest in the day-time' (K-W test; $P = 0.1622$) and 'It was easy to relax and feel at home in the ward' (K-W test; $P = 0.2337$). But there were marked differences in the scores of the mothers in the three hospitals for the statement 'I needed more rest at night' (K-W test; $P = 0.0001$). It was therefore concluded that the main parameter operating within this factor was that related to the amount of rest at night.

A number of studies have shown that subjects deprived of the deeper stages of sleep rapidly become depressed and lethargic and lose their efficiency in carrying out their normal activities. They find it difficult to take in information, and have particular difficulty with learning and performing manual tasks. Studies of the effects of sleep is an integral and vital part of the 24-hour biological cycle (Weinmann, 1981).

It is therefore not surprising to find that the 54 mothers whom the midwives described as being unduly distressed about feeding their babies in the postnatal ward, recorded significantly lower scores for the rest factor six weeks later (M-W test; P = 0.0244) (see Table 6.10).

Altogether 116 mothers (41.6 per cent of the total sample) had low scores on this factor, and those who were distressed about feeding accounted for almost half of them.

Important differences were found in the incidence of distress in feeding in the three hospitals, which provides further evidence of the relationship between lack of sleep and feeding difficulties. The mothers in hospital 2 scored significantly higher levels of satisfaction with the rest in hospital factor (K-W test; P = 0.0030) and the incidence of distress in feeding was significantly lower in this hospital than in the other two (chi-square = 12.972767; 4 d.f.; P = 0.0116). The self-image in feeding scores of mothers in hospital 2 were also significantly higher than those of mothers in the other hospitals (K-W test; P = 0.0223). There were no differences in the parity of the mothers in the three hospitals which might have accounted for these differences in the incidence of distress in feeding, nor were there any significant differences in anxiety rating (EPI(N) scores) which might have contributed towards sleep disturbance. Details can be seen in Table 6.12.

Table 6.12:A comparison of the mother's EPI(N) scores and scores for rest in hospital, self-image in feeding, emotional well-being and satisfaction with motherhood in the three hospitals (Kruskall-Wallis one-way analysis of variance)

Factors	Hospital 1 (mean rank) scores; $n = 112$)	Hospital 2 (mean rank) scores; $n = 103$)	Hospital 3 (mean rank) scores; $n = 63$)
EPI(N)	132.4	135.6	136.4
		$x^2 = 0.1412$; $P = 0.9318$	
Rest in hospital	132.6	160.3	119.7
		$x^2 = 11.6465$; $P = 0.0030$	
Self-image in feeding	128.8	157.0	131.9
		$x^2 = 7.6025$; $P = 0.0223$	
Emotional well-being	145.6	142.4	126.0
		$x^2 = 2.5252$; $P = 0.2829$	
Satisfaction with motherhood	141.0	143.8	131.9
		$x^2 = 0.9089$; $P = 0.6348$	

The differences in the mothers' scores for the rest in hospital factor and the effect which lack of sleep had upon their self-image in feeding and distress in feeding their babies were due to the different policies about the rooming-in of mothers and babies which operated in the three maternity hospitals. Rooming-in is the term given to the practice of keeping mothers and babies together as much as possible, and it has arisen as a result of studies of maternal-child relationships. (Klaus *et al*, 1972; Kennell *et al*, 1974; Leiderman and Seashore, 1975). Many hospitals have adopted a policy of 24-hour rooming-in, believing that any separation of mother and baby must be harmful.

The evidence of lack of sleep and its effects arising from this study indicates that while the theoretical concepts behind rooming-in may be soundly based, the practice of it left much to be desired. Although the results of the studies listed above are frequently cited as a basis for 24-hour rooming-in, an examination of the major publication by Klaus and Kennell (1982) reveals a recommendation that the baby should be kept at the mother's bedside for long periods in the daytime.

Hospital 2 had such a policy operating. For the first two days after delivery the babies were kept by their mothers' bedsides during the day from the time of the first feed in the morning until approximately 10 pm when they were taken into the ward nursery unless the mother particularly wanted her baby to remain with her during the night. They were then brought to their mothers for feeding during the night. On the third day the mothers were invited to have their babies with them throughout the 24 hours if they wished. The majority of them (69 per cent) went home during the third day, and many of those who remained, elected to continue the previous pattern of the baby sleeping in the nursery and being brought to them for feeding. As a result there were very few babies in the ward during the night.

In hospitals 1 and 3 the policy was that the babies were cared for in the ward nursery for the first night after delivery and then remained at the mother's bedside 24 hours a day. There were numerous complaints about the policies of rooming-in by the mothers in the hospitals concerned. It was not unusual for mothers to have their babies left with them throughout the first night after delivery.

One mother recalled that after several hours in labour her baby had been born in the early hours of the morning. That same night the baby was left by her bedside. All that night she cried continuously; no-one came to see if I needed any help.

> I felt so distraught...and was so tired I was afraid of dropping the baby. Finally at 2 am I had to get up and ask if someone would look after my baby so that I could get some sleep.

Another mother was put in a four-bedded ward with three antenatal mothers who had been admitted for rest.

> I was in a ward with three expectant mothers and I was the only one with a baby, so at his every whimper I was awake so that he wouldn't wake the others. After three days and nights with very little sleep I asked if the baby could go into the nursery just so I could get some sleep, but I was told the nursery was full with newborn babies.

It should be remembered that these comments were written by mothers six weeks after they had gone home from hospital, and they indicate the strong feelings mothers had about this matter. They also illustrate poor management of care by midwives on night duty, some of whom said that hospital policy did not allow them to take the babies out of the wards at night.

Lack of sleep is a frequent complaint of hospital patients, who find it difficult to settle in a strange environment and are disturbed by noise and lights. Disturbance is even more likely in any ward with newborn babies crying during the night. In a study of feeding and crying patterns of the newborn, Bernal (1972) noted that there was a peak of crying between midnight and 6 am. Many surveys of maternal satisfaction with postnatal care reveal a high degree of complaint about the lack of sleep caused by rooming-in policies. Clayton (1979) found that 47 per cent of the mothers in a modern maternity hospital complained of too little sleep because of rooming-in, and a study of postnatal care by Filshie et *al* (1981) found that 81 per cent of mothers nursed in four-bedded wards complained of lack of sleep. The 'That's Life' survey (Boyd and Sellers, 1982) collected the opinions of 6,000 self-elected mothers and found that many women did not want the baby to be with them throughout the night, but particularly liked the arrangement where babies stayed in the nursery at night and mothers were woken to feed them. A comparative study by Cox (1974) found that 40 per cent of the mothers whose babies stayed with them during the night from 48 hours after the birth complained of too little sleep. In a controlled study in the USA, Draramraj et *al* (1981) found that although certain groups of mothers certainly desired and appreciated 24-hour rooming-in, this opinion was by no means universal and that the factors which influenced the mothers' choice of whether to room-in or not varied among different groups of mothers. Cox and Draramraj both concluded that maternal choice should be the deciding factor in the matter.

It is unfortunate that in spite of all the evidence that mothers find 24-hour rooming-in troublesome, many maternity hospitals still practise the policy in a routine and indiscriminate manner.

The effects which conflicting advice and lack of sleep in hospital had upon the mothers' self-image and emotional well-being, uphold the second hypothesis that the way in which postnatal care is provided by midwives will affect the mother's emotional response to the changes which follow the birth of a child.

Satisfaction with motherhood - an enriching factor

The results discussed thus far in this chapter show how a mother's postnatal emotional well-being is affected by her personality and by a number of other stresses which make her vulnerable to emotional distress. There was, however, a third parameter in this interactive process and this had the effect of enriching the emotional response of the mother in such a way that she was enabled to overcome many of the difficulties which beset her. This parameter was the mother's satisfaction with motherhood, which was an outgoing emotion directed towards the baby rather than a reflection of the mother's internal emotional state.

Satisfaction with motherhood was measured by the mother's score on the satisfaction with motherhood factor - the second to emerge from the factor analysis of the emotional well-being questionnaire. This factor contained five statements which expressed the mother's feelings towards her baby. The possible range of scores was from 5 to 25, and the actual range of scores recorded by the mothers was from 14 to 25, with a mean average of 20.656 and a standard deviation of 2.410. This range of scores indicates the very positive pattern of scoring for this factor.

Only three mothers (1.1 per cent) recorded a score of 14 (equal to a mean average of less than 2.8 per statement), and these women were considered to have low satisfaction with motherhood; 77 mothers (27.6 per cent) scored between 15 and 19 (equal to a mean average of 3-3.95 per statement), and this group was classed as having moderate satisfaction with motherhood. The remaining 199 mothers (71.3 per cent) recorded scores of 20 or more (equal to a mean average of at least four per statement) and were considered to have very high satisfaction with motherhood.

A positive relationship was found between the mother's satisfaction with motherhood and her emotional well-being scores, the details of which can be seen in Table 6.13.

Table 6.13:EWB scores compared with scores for satisfaction with motherhood

(a)   Kruskall-Wallis one-way analysis of variance

Satisfaction with motherhood	EWB	
	n	Mean rank score
Low scores	3	33.8
Moderate scores	77	124.7
High scores	199	147.5

$x^2 = 9.7071;\ P = 0.0078$

(b)   Spearman rank correlation

Satisfaction with motherhood of mothers in:	n	EWB Spearman rank correlation	Significance
Hospital 1	112	0.3532	$P = 0.001$
Hospital 2	104	0.5557	$P = 0.001$
Hospital 3	63	-0.1650	Not signifgicant

Although the small number in the low satisfaction group is likely to have distorted the results of the one-way analysis of variance, analysis by Spearman rank correlation confirmed that there was a significant relationship between the scores for satisfaction with motherhood and emotional well-being of the 216 mothers in hospitals 1 and 2. This relationship was further confirmed by multiple regression analysis of the total sample, which will be discussed later.

As the overwhelming majority of mothers expressed high satisfaction with motherhood it would seem that the mother's joy and delight in her baby made a positive contribution to her emotional well-being, boosting her morale and enriching the adjustment process. Further analysis was therefore undertaken in order to identify any events or factors which might increase or decrease the degree of satisfaction with motherhood. A number of interesting facts were revealed.

Satisfaction with motherhood six weeks after the birth was found to be closely linked to the mother's reported feelings immediately after the birth of her baby, and those who fed their baby within an hour of the birth scored much more positive birth feelings and higher levels of satisfaction with motherhood six weeks later. Further analysis showed that these feelings were not influenced by those factors which had an adverse effect upon the mother's emotional well-being, and this suggests that they are a powerful and stable emotion.

Factors which did not affect satisfaction with motherhood

The degree of trait anxiety in the maternal personality - which had such a marked effect on her emotional well-being, self-confidence, and perception of hospital care and family support - did not affect satisfaction with motherhood (see Table 6.14).

Table 6.14:EPI(N) scores compared with scores for satisfaction with motherhood

Satisfaction with motherhood	EPI(N)	
	n	Mean rank scores
Low scores	3	143.0
Moderate scores	75	128.1
High scores	190	136.9
		$x^2 = 0.7350;\ P = 0.6925$

Mothers who had a low score for self-image in feeding, and those who were seen to be distressed about their infants whilst in hospital, did not score any less satisfaction with motherhood than other mothers (see Tables 6.9 and 6.10).

Rooming-in practices

Although lack of rest in hospital was related to the patterns of rooming-in of babies and mothers, and had an effect on emotional well-being, it did not have a similar effect on satisfaction with motherhood (see Table 6.9) and there were no significant differences in the satisfaction with motherhood of the mothers in the three different hospitals (see Table 6.12). This indicates that the practice of putting babies in the nursery at night did not have a detrimental effect upon the developing relationship between the mother and her baby.

Infant feeding

Mothers who bottlefed their infants did not record any less satisfaction with motherhood than breastfeeding mothers, and there was no evidence that the mother's age or parity had any significant effect upon her satisfaction with motherhood (see Table 6.15).

Table 6.15:Scores for satisfaction with motherhood classified by age, parity, and choice of feeding method

Variable	Satisfaction with motherhood	
	n	Mean rank scores
Age of mother		
17-20 years	31	146.4
21-29 years	164	135.3
30-39 years	84	146.8
K-W test:	$x^2 = -1.3637$; $P = 0.5057$	
Parity		
Primigravidae	98	144.2
Multiparae	179	136.1
M-W test:	$z = 0.8097$; $P = 0.4181$	
Choice of feeding method		
Breast	161	141.0
Bottle	112	131.2
M-W test:	$z = 1.0238$; $P = 0.3059$	

Factors associated with different levels of satisfaction with motherhood

Links between satisfaction with motherhood scores and mothers reported feelings at birth

A highly significant relationship was found between the mother's reported feelings immediately after delivery and her satisfaction with motherhood six weeks later (Table 6.16). The details of the interview in which the mother recorded these feelings are given in Chapter 4.

It can be seen in Table 6.16 that the six mothers who said that they were 'disappointed' and the 19 who said that they felt 'too tired to care' scored the lowest levels of satisfaction with motherhood, and the highest level of satisfaction was recorded by the 71 mothers who said that they had felt 'gloriously happy' immediately after the birth of the baby.

Table 6.16: Scores for satisfaction with motherhood compared with mothers' reported feelings after delivery (Kruskall-Wallis one-way analysis of variance)

	Satisfaction with motherhood[2]	
Feelings after delivery[1]	*n*	*Mean rank score*
Disappointed	6	76.3
Too tired to care	19	105.3
Relieved	82	125.9
Tired and happy	83	110.7
Gloriously happy	71	172.2

$X^2 = 33.4957$; $P = 0.0001$

[1] Recorded within 24-36 hours of the birth. Fourteen mothers gave no definite answer and are not included·
[2] Recorded 6-8 weeks after the birth.

There is some evidence that mothers who were highly motivated towards motherhood before delivery scored more positive feelings immediately after the baby's birth, and that mothers who fed their newborn infants during the first hour after delivery also recalled more positive feelings. During the antenatal interview 67 women had expressed their eager anticipation of becoming mothers, some of them for the second or third time, and these women later expressed much more positive feelings after the birth.There was no evidence that the type of labour or delivery affected the mother's feelings immediately afterwards (see Table 6.17).

Table 6.17: Scores for birth feelings classified by type of labour and delivery

	Birth feelings	
Variable	*n*	*Mean rank score*
Type of labour		
Spontaneous	121	131.6
Induced	97	148.4
Active Management	58	136.3
		$X^2 = 2.6064; P = 0.2717$
Type of delivery		
Normal	194	137.7
Forceps	49	133.1
Breech	4	161.8
Caesarian Section	29	149.8
		$X^2 = 1.2556; P = 0.7397$

It appears that the mother's attention immediately after the birth was centred upon her newborn infant and her feelings towards him or her, rather than the events of labour and delivery which had resulted in the birth. It is therefore not surprising to find that the giving and receiving of a feed enhanced the mother's pleasure in her achievement, and it could be argued that the pleasure of giving a feed made a difference to the mothers recollection of her feelings immediately after the birth.

Effect on satisfaction with motherhood of feeding the baby in the first hour after delivery

Mothers who fed their babies during the first hour after delivery recalled more positive feelings at that time and the highest levels of satisfaction with motherhood six weeks later (see Table 6.18).

Table 6.18: Scores for birth feelings and satisfaction with motherhood classified by time of first feed to infant (Mann-Whitney U test corrected for ties)

(a)   Birth feelings

Time of first feed	Birth feelings (24 hours after birth)	
	n	Mean rank score
Within 1 hour of birth	112	153.3
More than 1 hour after birth	164	129.8
	$Z = 2.2769; P = 0.0228$	

(b)   Satisfaction with motherhood

Time of first feed	Satisfaction with motherhood (6 weeks after birth)	
	n	Mean rank score
Within 1 hour of birth	113	151.6
More than 1 hour after birth	165	131.2
	$Z = 2.0921; P = 0.0364$	

A number of studies have focused upon the contact between the mother and her baby during the first hour after delivery, and have demonstrated the beneficial effect which a period of mutual physical contact has upon the developing maternal-child relationship. When a baby is held in the *en face* position he or she is able to gaze into the mother's eyes, and this creates a deep bond between them. It has also been observed that when mothers are left alone with their newborn infants they follow a particular pattern of exploring the baby's body (Klaus *et al*, 1972, 1975; Leiderman and Seashore, 1975; Klaus and Kennell, 1970, 1976, 1982). The giving of a feed allows a mother to have a period of uninterrupted time with her baby during the first hour after the birth, and appears to assume a pivotal position between her experience of labour and delivery and her outward and infant-directed feelings of joy and satisfaction with motherhood.

It might be supposed that mothers who had a difficult delivery would be less likely to feed their babies, but this was not so. Of the women who had a forceps delivery, 40 per cent fed their babies during the first hour compared with 45 per cent of those who had a normal delivery. Two of the four women who had a breech delivery fed their babies, and three of the mothers who had a caesarean section under epidural analgesia fed their babies whilst still in the operating theatre. It would appear that whether or not a mother fed her baby during the first hour after birth depended upon her choice of breast or bottlefeeding, and upon the management of care in the delivery suite. There is also considerable evidence that younger women and those from lower social classes were less likely to be given an opportunity to feed their baby, and that those who had received Pethidine in labour were also less likely to feed their babies. The details of the analysis can be seen in Tables 6.19 and 6.20.

Table 6.19: Factors/events affecting mothers who fed or who did not feed their babies within one hour of birth

Note: All the hospitals had a policy for putting baby to breast as soon as possible after birth

	Mother fed baby		Mother did not feed baby		Total	
	n	%	*n*	%	*n*	%
Total sample	109	40.6	163	59.4	272	100
1. Type of labour						
Spontaneous	57	46.3	66	53.7	123	100
Induced	37	38.1	60	61.9	97	100
Augmented	19	32.8	39	67.2	58	100

n/s; chi-square; p = .1825

	Mother fed baby		Mother did not feed baby		Total	
2. Type of delivery						
Normal	88	45.1	107	54.9	195	100
Forceps	20	40.0	30	60.0	50	100
Breech/Caesarian*	5	15.2	28	84.8	33	100

*sig; chi-square; p = .01 **

	Mother fed baby		Mother did not feed baby		Total	
3. Type of pain relief						
Pethidine or Epidural	78	37.3	129	62.3	207	100
Nitrous oxide only and/or no other form of pain relief	34	63.0	20	37.0	54	100

sig; chi-square; p = .0001

* This result due to small number of caesarians; not significant for main sample of normal/ forceps cases.

Table 6.20: Factors/events affecting mothers who fed or who did not feed their babies within one hour of birth

Note: All the hospitals had a policy for putting baby to breast as soon as possible after birth

	Mother fed baby		Mother did not feed baby		Total	
	n	%	n	&	n	&
Total sample	109	40.6	163	59.4	272	100
4. Feeding method chosen						
Breast	93	58.1	67	41.9	160	100
Bottle	16	14.3	96	85.7	112	100

sig; chi-square; p = .0001

	n	%	n	&	n	&
5. Age of mother						
17-20 years	5	12.9	27	87.1	31	100
21-29 years	70	42.9	93	57.1	153	100
30-39 years	39	45.9	46	54.1	84	100

sig; chi-square; p = .01

	n	%	n	&	n	&
6. Social class of mother						
Classes 1 and 2	44	51.8	41	48.2	85	100
Class 3 non-manual	20	51.3	19	48.7	39	100
Class 3 manual	25	36.8	43	63.2	68	100
Classes 4 and 5	19	26.0	52	74.0	73	100
Unclassified	4	36.4	7	63.6	11	100

sig; chi-square; p = .01

During the first hour, 113 mothers (40.5 per cent of the total sample) fed their babies, and of these 107 breastfed their babies and six bottlefed. All the hospitals had policies which said that mothers should be encouraged to put the baby to the breast as soon as possible after birth, the main purpose behind the policy being the need for the stimulation of lactation in mothers who intended to breastfeed. The enrichment of the maternal-child relationship which suckling a baby also brings seemed to be overlooked. However, even though such policies were in existence, it was found that 76 of the 183 mothers who had elected to breastfeed did not put their babies to the breast at this time.

As the study did not include observing the birth of the baby, it is not possible to ascertain all the events which led to a mother feeding or not feeding her baby. However, there is some evidence to suggest that the more articulate mothers were given a greater opportunity to feed their babies. Although allowance must be made for the social class differences in the choice of breast or bottlefeeding, it is notable that 60 per cent of those who fed their babies came from social classes 1, 2 and 3n/m, and only 40 per cent from social classes 3m, 4 and 5. Mothers aged between 21 and 29 years formed 62 per cent of those who fed their babies. Ten mothers aged under 20 elected to breastfeed but only three of them fed their babies during the first hour after the birth.

Attention must also be called to the needs of mothers who chose to bottlefeed, as it is these women who were most deprived of the opportunity which the giving of a feed provided for the mother and her baby to be left alone together. At the time when the research was carried out it was quite rare for a woman to be offerred an opportunity to bottlefeed her baby, mainly because no-one had thought about it. It is in the giving and receiving of a feed that maternal-child relationships are enriched, and it is to be regretted that mothers who choose to bottlefeed are rarely given an opportunity to do so shortly after the baby's birth. Indeed it may be some time before mother and baby enjoy a feed together in the postnatal ward. The same en face position that the baby automatically assumes when held to suckle at the breast can also be achieved when the baby is held in the mother's arms to bottlefeed.

As the giving of a feed was associated with positive feelings immediately after delivery and increased satisfaction with motherhood six weeks later, it is likely that careful management of post-delivery care, which ensures that every mother and baby spend a period of time together, would enrich the experience of motherhood and, by its reinforcement of the mother's feelings towards her baby, could make a positive contribution to her emotional well-being.

Conclusions

The results of this study show that maternal emotional well-being measured six weeks after the birth of the baby was significantly affected by or associated with three interacting sets of factors. Maternal and family factors made up a framework which made some women vulnerable to distress. The effects of anxiety can be seen throughout the postnatal period, marital tension and other life-stress events also played their part. Another set of factors surround the birth and the mother's feelings at that time, and whether or not she was able to feed or have unhurried contact with her baby. The influence of these birth events is seen in the separate parameter of satisfaction with motherhood. The third set of factors is linked to events of postnatal self-image in feeding, which was eroded by conflicting advice and lack of sleep in hospital.

In order to determine the degree to which these different factors combined together to affect postnatal emotional outcome, a further analysis was undertaken using multiple regression. This technique examines the degree to which differences in a group of significant variables affect the dependent variable (Stopher and Meyburg, 1979).

Which factors made the most impact upon emotional well-being?

A number of analyses were carried out, using both the stepwise and direct forms of regression. The full range of maternal scores for emotional well-being were tested against the mother's anxiety score on the Eysenck Personality Inventory (EPI(N) score), the birth feelings scores, all the postnatal care factor scores, the satisfaction with motherhood scores and the mother's perception of her baby's progress measured by her scores on the Broussard-type scale.

The highest multiple regression score (multiple R = 0.70746) was obtained when the combined effect of the group of factors shown in Table 6.21 was analysed. The factors are listed in the table in the order in which they are shown by the regression to have had a predictive effect upon emotional outcome.

Table 6.21: Multiple regression analysis of major factors related to postnatal emotional well-being

Dependent variable: emotional well-being

Mean response	78.34601	Standard deviation	11.45078
Multiple *R*	0.70746	Analysis of variance	DF
R square	0.50049	Regression	8
Adjusted *R* square	0.48476	Residual	254
S.D.	8.21938	Coefficient of variability	10.5%

F = 31.81283; Level of significance = 0.0001

Variable	*B* coefficient	S.E. of *B*	F/Significance
Family support (six weeks post-partum)	1.2460546	0.24199185	25.513844/ 0.0001
Self-confidence (1-2 weeks post-partum)	1.1396136	0.31803888	12.839698/ 0.0001
Broussard-type score (6 weeks post-partum)	1.1197801	0.58280626	3.6916206/ 0.056
Self-image in feeding	0.67895392	0.25635193	7.0146730/ 0.009
Family support (1-2 weeks post-partum)	0.67188137	0.24073798	7.7892556/ 0.006
EPI(N) score (36 weeks pregnant)	-0.59274737	0.12135500	23.857445/ 0.0001
Satisfaction with motherhood (6 weeks post-partum)	0.52256611	0.22479123	5.4041040/ 0.021
Ward atmosphere (1 week post-partum)	0.31435893	0.16352195	3.6957235/ 0.056

The consistent relationship between personality and emotional well-being is seen in the presence of the EPI(N) scores and in four other factors which also related to the mother's degree of anxiety. The EPI(N) score which was recorded approximately four weeks before the baby was born is placed sixth in relation to the mother's emotional well-being when her baby was six weeks old. The degree of anxiety in a mother's personality also affected her ability to relax and feel at home in the postnatal ward (eighth in order), her perception of family support (fifth in order) and her self-confidence when she first came home (second in order). Its continuing effect is seen in the first factor listed in the predictive order, which was the mother's perception of the quality of the support she was receiving from her family at the time when she filled in the questionnaire.

The less anxious women were coping quite well and felt that the help they were receiving was sufficient for their needs, but the scores of the distressed women constituted a cry for help. They were not yet able to cope alone and felt that they needed more help than they were receiving. Although the results show that anxiety played a large part in their perceptions, these scores also call into question the assumption that a woman 'ought' to be able to cope with all the demands of the household by the time her baby is six weeks old.

The remaining factors listed were not related to the mother's personality but arose from her feelings towards her baby and about her own competence in mothering, and were affected to a certain degree by the care she received from midwives.

The Broussard-type score was listed third in the predictive order and its relationship to both emotional well-being and satisfaction with motherhood suggest that it was a powerful indicator of the mother's feelings and perceptions six weeks after the birth of the baby. The mother's score on this scale was closely associated with her score for self-image in feeding which is fourth in the predictive order and which was affected by stress in the postnatal ward.

Satisfaction with motherhood, which acted as a boost to the mother's emotional state, was listed seventh, indicating the significance of its contribution to the adjustment process.

The results of the study and the interaction of significant factors shown in the results of the multiple regression analysis upheld both hypotheses. The mother's personality and the quality of her family and social support certainly affected her response to the changes which resulted from the birth of her baby, and the way that midwives cared for the mother during the postnatal period also had a significant effect upon her well-being.

CHAPTER 7

"Loading the Dice": Interaction of Personal Needs, Stresses and Support Systems

The results of the study show how the 279 women in the sample reacted to the experience and demands of motherhood, and the way that their reactions were influenced by the interaction of a number of factors, some of which could be classified as fixed, e.g. trait anxiety and life-stress events, and some mainly care factors, which were alterable. Each of these factors had their own part to play, as well as exerting an interactive and cumulative effect.

The results revealed two distinct but related measures of outcome: emotional well-being and satisfaction with motherhood; and demonstrated that factors which affected one did not affect the other. Therefore it seems that there is more than one set of influences upon a woman's reactions to motherhood.

How did the mothers fare?
Most of the mothers in the sample were coping quite well six weeks after the birth; 31 scored high levels of emotional well-being, feeling very happy and coping well, 194 scored moderate but satisfactory levels of emotional well-being, and were coping quite well although they would have liked a bit more help. The remaining 54 had low scores and were unhappy, feeling overwhelmed with things, needed more help than they were receiving and some were depressed. This is sad, and it is no real comfort to note that the percentage of the sample who had low scores is consistent with the percentage found in other studies of postnatal depression.

However, when we consider all the many changes and demands that mother faces: loss of control over lifestyle which is now completely overtaken by the needs of a small baby, and the lack of sleep which goes along with it, perhaps we should ask why it is only 20 per cent!

Part of the answer lies in the way that the joy and delight which parents feel in their new baby, and the fulfilment of dreams which he or she brings, more than compensates for the upheaval and demands. The majority of the mother's in the sample recorded high levels of satisfaction with motherhood; 190 mothers scored high satisfaction and many of them wrote about their joy and delight, another 75 scored more moderate scores but still within the realm of satisfaction and pleasure. Only three mothers, all of whom were bordering on depression, scored low levels of satisfaction with motherhood and they also had low scores on the Broussard scale.

Interactive framework of reactions to motherhood

The main significant factors and their interaction are shown in Figures 7.1 and 7.2. For the sake of clarity, fixed variables (antecedent and life events) are shown separately in Figure 7.1, and other factors, most of which are alterable in 7.2.

Fig. 7.1:Antecedent factors related to emotional well-being and satisfaction with motherhood six weeks after the birth

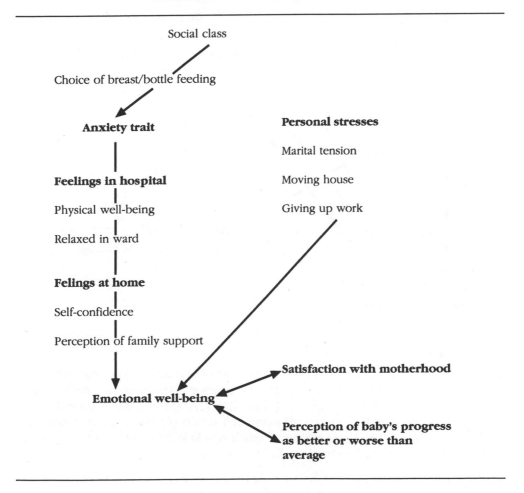

Figure 7.1 shows those maternal and family factors which most influenced emotional well-being throughout the postnatal period.

Fig. 7.2: Other factors related to emotional well-being and satisfaction with motherhood six weeks after the birth

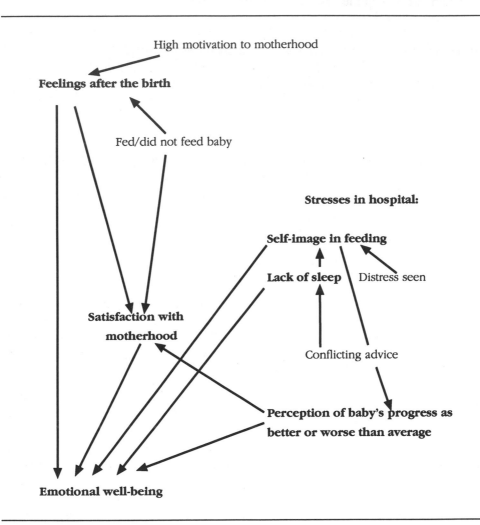

Trait anxiety

The effect of trait anxiety were identified by Tod (1964) and Pitt (1968). However, Kumar and Robson (1984) did not find it to be a factor when emotional well-being in mothers was measured at three months post-delivery, suggesting that its impact passes with time. Some new information also emerged which is particularly interesting for maternity services. The choice of infant feeding was linked to trait anxiety, with more anxious women choosing to bottlefeed.

Personal stresses

The presence or absence of life-stress factors is also found in the results of other studies, especially marital tension (Brown and Harris, 1978; Paykel 1980; Oakley, 1980; Kumar and Robson, 1984; O'Hara, 1983; Stein *et al*, 1989), and moving house (Paykel, 1980).

The similarities between the results shown in Figure 7.1 and other major studies from the field of psychiatry or psychology based studies add weight and validation to this midwifery-focused study.

The factors shown in Figure 7.1 seem to be mainly fixed. Trait anxiety was closely linked to the mother's feeling of well-being and confidence, showing clearly the impact of this antecedent factor upon the coping processes. It might be possible to dissuade parents from moving house just before a baby is born, but there is little that care-givers can do to change the other factors. However, we should not forget that becoming a mother is a peak life experience (Erikson, 1963) and that a good experience can boost a woman's confidence in herself to a considerable degree.

Figure 7.2 shows a different group of factors. These fell into two main groups, both of which were affected to some degree by care factors, which gives us our first clue that there are some factors in reactions to motherhood which are not fixed but can be used to enhance and strengthen women. There seem to be two influences here, one of which may be fixed. The first group links the mother's feelings after birth, her satisfaction with motherhood and the Broussard score, with the emotional well-being score. There is some link between the mother's expressed high motivation to motherhood recorded in late pregnancy and very positive feelings after the birth which suggest that this reflects the mother's deep inner feelings about having this baby. It was, however, influenced by care factors, with those who fed the baby scoring much more positive feelings and higher levels of satisfaction with motherhood six weeks later. This suggests that this factor is picking up something of the concept of fixed and alterable influences upon the attachment process which are discussed by Klaus and Kennell (1976, 1982) and confirmed by Siegel (1982).

The second group of factors certainly reflect the alterable care factor. One of the surprising things about these data is that although one might have expected that the mother's self-image in feeding and the care factors which affected it, would have some impact upon her satisfaction with motherhood, this is not the case. These factors affected her emotional well-being which indicates how the presence or absence of care-related stress affected the coping process.

The results clearly underline the usefulness of the coping process as a model, which helps us to understand the different aspects of adjustment and to harness that understanding in expanding the knowledge which all care-givers require if they are to provide women with a coordinated and sensitive pattern of care. Such care must, in its planning and delivery, accord as much importance to the emotional and spiritual well-being of mothers and babies, as it does to their physical well-being.

Which factors made the most difference?

Figures 7.1 and 7.2 illustrate the way the different factors "fitted" together, but it is in the multiple regression analysis (Table 6.21 Chapter 6) that we can see the combination of factors which made most difference to the emotional well-being of the women in the study. If a woman scored badly on all the eight factors shown below, then she would be almost certain to be distressed, whilst those with high scores on each factor would fall within the very happy and well-adjusted group, while most would have a combination of good and poorer scores. If the poorer scores could be improved, then the outcome would be better. Although some of the factors listed below are clearly linked to anxiety which was a fixed variable which "loaded the dice", others were affected by care practices, which could be changed. Good scores on these factors could counterbalance the effect of antecedent and stress factors.

These factors, which were most associated with different levels of maternal emtional well-being six weeks after the birth of the baby, are listed again below. The order indicates the strength of the cumulative effect of each within the combination shown and the degree to which each factor is predictive of the outcome.

How the dice were loaded

*1.   Perception of family support six weeks post-delivery.
*2.   Mother's reported self-confidence when she first returned home with the baby (60 per cent on or before third day; 23 per cent 3-7 days, 17 per cent 7+ days).
3.   Mother's rating of her baby's progress as better or worse than "average" (Broussard scale) six weeks post-delivery.
4.   Mother's self-image in feeding her baby during her stay in hospital (60 per cent 1-3 days, 23 per cent 3-7 days, 17 per cent 7+ days).
*5.   Perception of family support when mother first came home with baby.
*6.   Trait anxiety score on the Eysenck personality Inventory measured four weeks before the birth.
7.   Satisfaction with motherhood six weeks after delivery.
*8.   Reactions to ward atmosphere during hospital stay.

It should be remembered that in undertaking the multiple regression analysis, the full range of scores on each factor for the whole sample of 279 women were compared with the full range of scores for emotional well-being.

Fixed factors: effect of personality as an antecedent factor
In the list above, those scores marked with an asterisk were shown in other analyses to be closely linked levels of trait anxiety measured by the EPI (Eysenck and Eysenck, 1968) (see Tables 6.3, 6.5, 6.6, Chapter 6). This does not mean, however, that these results relate only to anxious women. The sample scored are range of scores on the EPI indicating high, moderate and low levels of anxiety. This factor predisposed the woman's reactions via her personality, with less anxious women feeling more confident than the high anxious women.

Although these factors show the influence of anxiety as a predisposing or antecedent factor, the regression shows that their level of significance reduces the further they are from the time when the emotional well-being questionnaire was completed. It is likely, therefore, that they reflect the mother's initial degree of confidence which would be affected by her degree of anxiety, and then be further influenced by what happened as she began to cope with the responsibilities of mothering.

These factors clearly support hypothesis 1, and suggest a means of identifying anxious or stressed mothers in order to provide increased support. There was some evidence that both hospital and community midwives recognized the stress which the mother's felt at different times of the puerperium.

The Broussard score

This factor, which was placed high at number 3, was not influenced by anxiety, nor were care factors identified which might have had some impact. As it was completed at the same time as the emotional well-being questionnaire, it is likely that the mother's state at that time was the most important influence. Indeed it was designed by Broussard (1971) to be used as a screening tool to identify women who were distressed or not coping with their babies. The main significance of the Broussard score lies in its relationship with both the emotional well-being and satisfaction with motherhood scores. The most significant link was with emotional well-being (p=0.0005) rather than satisfaction with motherhood (P=0.0078). The mother's age, parity or social class did not have any bearings on this score, although multiparae had higher mean scores. The choice of infant feeding had no bearing either, nor did feeding the baby in the first hour after delivery. There was however a significant relationship with the mother's self-image in feeding score (p=0.0064) which suggests that, for some mothers, uncertainty and difficulties in feeding in the very first days after delivery were not resolved with time and may have had a bad influence on attachment between the mother and her baby. However, evidence for this is very tentative. The Broussard score, however, does have value as an indicator that a mother needs extra help, and could be used as an early warning of potential problems. There is evidence from a number of studies that early intervention can be effective in reducing the incidence of postnatal depression (Holden *et al*, 1989; Elliott *et al*, 1983; Cox, 1989).

Alterable factors

Two other factors were not affected by the mother's personality or life-stress events. Self-image in feeding was placed fourth and satisfaction with motherhood seventh. Although these were completed at the same time as the emotional well-being score, other data showed that they were affected by a number of care practices events which were recorded in the next few days. These will be reviewed later in the chapter.

As well as upholding the second hypothesis and Caplan's (1969, 1976) view of the importance of support systems, they also provide some of the most valuable information about care practices which enhance or reduce a woman's strengths and joys.

But, the results did not indicate that the major patterns of organizing maternity care, e.g. management of labour, early discharge, length of visiting by community midwives, directly affected reaction to motherhood. Instead it was a more subtle set of care patterns and events which arose from individual approach and attitudes of midwives in both hospital and community services. These were themselves affected by the culture of the hospital organization and possibly pressure of work. Some of these issues will be reviewed later in the chapter.

Changing the balance - creating a supportive environment

The results of the study show how adjustment to motherhood is influenced by the balance between several factors, each of which interact with each other in a complex and dynamic process.

Although the outcome of the coping process is strongly influenced by personality, previous experiences, the attitudes and expectations of family and peers and the way a person reacts to change is the result of the interaction between personal needs and attributes, the volume of stress to which an individual is exposed and the quality of the supportive environment which surrounds that individual (Lazarus, 1966, 1969; Caplan, 1969; Caplan and Killelia, 1976; Derlega and Janda, 1978).

Potential for influencing the outcome

The results of the studies demonstrate that the supportive environment provided by the midwifery services did indeed make a difference to the interactive framework and its effect upon mother's emotional well-being and satisfaction with motherhood.

The potential of this interactive framework is perhaps best illustrated by the story of Janet who was one of the mothers who gave birth in Hospital 3. Her story which is reproduced just as she wrote it on the back of her postnatal questionnaire shows how she had many problems which made her vulnerable to emotional distress, and how these were counterbalanced by Janet's own sense of humour and by the sensitive care of her obstetrician, the help of her husband and a close friend and by the care of a "smashing midwife".

Anxiety

Janet was a married woman of 28 years, pregnant for the second time. The pregnancy was not planned. Her first child was a boy of eight years old, who had been born by caesarean section. In the antenatal interview Janet had expressed great fear about the possibility of another caesarean section. Her anxiety score on the Eysenck Personality Inventory was high and her extroversion/introversion score was average.

Stress factors

Janet's husband had recently become unemployed from his job as a truck driver. Janet had been working as a bakery operative until six weeks before the baby was born.

The family was experiencing considerable financial problems which had begun when Janet's husband lost his job, and had not been improved by a serious fire which had damaged their council flat four months previously. This had been due to faulty wiring, for which the council had taken responsibility. However, the council had told Janet and her husband that the redecoration of the flat could not be undertaken for at least six months. As the new baby was due before that time, the couple had undertaken the work themselves, but the council then refused to meet the costs because they said that Janet and her husband should have waited for them to do it. This argument had not been resolved by the time the baby was actually born, and Janet and her husband had got into arrears with the rent.

Obstetric problems

Janet was allowed to go into normal labour in the hope that she could deliver her baby vaginally, but this did not prove possible, and after eight hours of labour she gave birth to another son, Daniel, by caesarean section under general anaesthetic. The baby's condition at birth was excellent. Janet chose to bottlefeed her baby and did not give him a feed herself until he was over 24 hours old.

Postnatal care

The postnatal ward staff noted that Janet seemed to be distressed about feeding her baby and considered that this was due to discomfort after the caesarean section. They also noted that she was tearful, not sleeping well, and somewhat irritable during her stay in hospital.

Janet comments on her hospital care:

> It is difficult to answer about being fit and well, because I did feel well really, except that I had a terrible problem with wind. None of the nurses or doctors seemed to know how bad it was; they kept giving me some white stuff which did no good at all. It was only when I couldn't stand it any longer after two whole days without sleep because of the pain, that they took any notice, and they only took notice because I was crying. They gave me some suppositories and they didn't work very well either. In the end I got rid of it myself with experience, bending up and down. The relief was so great I skipped back to bed. Other than that I felt perfectly well. The only other thing that spoiled my stay in hospital was the food - it was awful. I got my husband and sister to bring me in sandwiches because I was starving. And the rules over staying up and watching television. I think they aren't fair at all - they make you feel as though you are in prison or something, saying you've got to go to bed at a certain time. Hospital is boring enough so I think you should have something to look forward to even if it's only the late film.

Janet went home when the baby was seven days old. She writes about her experiences then:

After I arrived home I did find it difficult to rest, but with the help of my husband and a very good friend who lives around the corner I seemed to manage. My friend Pauline told me I looked very tired and so that I could sleep she took the baby for a whole day. It was the best sleep I had for a long time. Don't get me wrong, baby Daniel was very good, but I was conscious that he was there and that I must wake up every four hours for him. I'm still nervous now if he sleeps for a long time because I'm frightened of him dying from cot death and if anything happened to him now I don't know what I'd do. Some people have different ideas about letting babies sleep. The nurses say don't let him sleep longer than six hours, and older women I've talked to say let him sleep, he'll wake when he wants to, but I want him up - I'm not taking any chances.

The midwives who came to see me were marvellous, especially the one who came all the time. She used to ask me all about the baby and myself, and seemed really concerned. I really looked forward to her coming for a chat and advice. She never seemed to be in a hurry, she was a smashing lady. She seemed more like a mother to me and always told me off if she found I'd been doing housework. I didn't need to do anything at all, I had more than enough help, but I don't like putting on people.

She discusses how she feels now that Daniel is six weeks old:

In answer to number 7 [on the emotional well-being questionnaire] I do get upset easily, I don't know why. My husband says I snap at him for the least little thing but he says he understands. I also get weepy but mostly when I'm on my own.

I talk to the baby all the time. He's gorgeous and now he's talking back to me and saying agoo, and he's nearly always smiling. I'd do anything for him when he smiles and tries to talk back to me, he makes me feel all excited.

When my first baby was born, I was 19 years old and my husband was 18. I was very poorly having him and sure that if I ever had to have another section I would kill myself. When I found I was having another one with Daniel I told my husband to take the baby and leave me because I didn't think I'd live through it, but everything was fine. On my first baby the nurse took all my jewellery off me and put it in a brown envelope. I had bad dreams all during the operation, and I dreamt that my husband came to the hospital and all they gave him was this brown envelope, yet on this second operation they just covered my jewellery with plaster and I had no bad dreams.

The reason I mentioned our ages is because I think that we were too young to have a baby then. My husband never helped me hardly at all, he just didn't seem interested in the baby, yet this time he feeds the baby and always wakes up when he's crying. And he's even changed him a few times - one thing I thought he'd never do. In fact I'm very proud of him. As we've gotten older I think we've become more settled and going out doesn't bother us like it did nine years ago.

Sometimes I do feel that the baby doesn't belong to me. It's hard to get used to having a baby really after waiting eight years since my other little boy.

After my first baby when I went for the coil the doctor asked me if I wanted more babies, and as I really wanted a girl I said yes. He said that if I had the coil I would probably never conceive again but he didn't say why. Therefore I didn't have the coil and I was poorly on the pill. All that was left was the sheath and that kept bursting and I was frightened because I was told you had a bad time if you got pregnant that way. I think that had a lot do with feeling that my baby isn't mine is because I thought I would never have another, and with a caesarean one minute he's inside and the next he's out - you don't see him being born - so you don't feel he's yours at first. But both boys look so like their father that I know they're mine and I can see that they're mine.

I know that my baby knows that I love him by the way he looks at me and smiles - his eyes are full of love. If he wakes up crying in his pram and I call his name and go to him, he smiles and gets excited, because he knows I love him very much. I love kissing the back of his neck and feeling his bottom. I love when he is in the nude and I can feel his lovely warm body next to mine. His skin feels beautiful.

The lessons from Janet's story

It can be seen that there were a number of factors which 'loaded the dice' for Janet and made her a potential candidate for emotional distress.

The events of her previous pregnancy and caesarean section had left her with a great dread of repeating the experience. The pregnancy was unplanned, and Janet says that she was convinced she would die if she had another caesarean section. She recounts how young and immature she and her husband were at the time of the older boy's birth.

Janet had a high degree of anxiety trait in her personality and she and her husband had recently faced a number of stressful life-events. She did not feed Daniel until 24 hours after his birth, and she did not feel relaxed or at home in the hospital situation. These loading factors were counteracted by the kind of support Janet received, and the growing maturity of Janet and her husband.

The obstetrician who cared for Janet was very sympathetic to her fears, and made every endeavour to enable Janet to have a vaginal delivery for her second baby. The trust which had grown between them enabled Janet to face the second operation and to find it an altogether different experience from the first. Her friend Pauline seemed to have had a great deal of common sense and stepped in with an offer of help at just the right moment.

It is obvious that Janet felt her community midwife cared about her as an individual, was unhurried, friendly and approachable: 'She seemed like a mother to me'.

Janet's story had a happy ending, and the way in which she wrote so fully about her experiences demonstrates the sense of satisfaction and achievement which the birth and mothering of Daniel brought to her, and through her to her whole family.

Her account of the help she received from Pauline and the midwife is a cameo of the effective helper described by Caplan (1969) and Weiss (1976). Both define effective support as that which enables the stressed individual to accept the helper as an ally, and which assures him or her that the helper's skill, time and understanding are available for as long as they are needed. The secret of success in being such a helper lies in the relationship which develops between the individual and the care-giver.

This has been widely demonstrated in the evidence given to the Winterton Committee (House of Commons, 1992) and recognized in the thrust to provide a key worker, who might be either a midwife, general practitioner or obstetrician who will provide continuity and unity of care for each individual woman throughout pregnancy, labour and postnatal care. (Ball *et al*, 1992; Department of Health, 1993). The purpose behind these initiatives are to reduce fragmentation of maternity care and to enable good relationships to flourish. It will be equally important to ensure that sensitive care practices are integrated within the objectives of each aspect of the maternity services, and not restricted to the personal attributes and skills of particular midwives, doctors and other staff.

Using the research findings to build a sensitive supportive framework

In the discussion which follows, fuller details are given of the data surrounding the two other factors which were shown in the analysis to have some influence upon emotional outcome but were not found to be linked to antecedent factors or life-stress events.

Self-image in feeding baby in first days after birth

The self-image in feeding factor score expressed the mother's retrospective assessment of how she had felt about herself when she embarked upon the feeding of her baby. It was not a measure of the quality of feeding support she felt she had from midwives, which was measured separately.

The factor was made up from the scores on the following statements.

•   Feeding my baby was a worry.
•   I needed more help in feeding my baby than I was given.
•   Other mothers seemed to manage better than I did.

The self-image in feeding score was listed fourth in the regression analysis, and it might have been supposed that the close relationship with emotional well-being was primarily due to the woman's emotional state when she completed both the emotional well-being questionnaire and the postnatal questionnaire six weeks after the birth. If this had been the case, however, one would have expected to find a statistically significant relationship with the satisfaction with motherhood factor, scored at the same time, and this was not the case (see Table 6.9). Other data also revealed that the mother's scores on this factor were linked to events and care factors in the hospital, and to the midwives observations recorded on the day each mother was discharged from hospital (see Table 6.10).

The significance of these care factors is increased when others which might have been expected to play a role are dismissed.

Self-image in feeding was not related to anxiety (p=0.1100), social class (p=0.9073), labour (p=0.6508) delivery or to the timing of the first feed to the baby (p = 0.6097). Neither was it related to the third day maternity blues (p=0.2908).

Age and parity and choice of feeding method

As might have been expected, younger mothers (p=0.01) and primigravidae (p=0.0003) had significantly lower scores. However, as age and parity were not a factor in emotional well-being six weeks later, it seems that many of this inexperienced group of mothers had gained a good deal of confidence in feeding by six weeks post-delivery.

There was a tentative link with the choice of feeding methods which was just at significance level (p=0.05). One might have assumed that this illustrated the early problems of establishing breastfeeding, but it was in fact the bottlefeeding women who had lower self-image in feeding. This raises questions about allocating help to mothers, most midwives emphasize the needs of breastfeeders and it can be easy to assume that bottlefeeding mothers do not need help. Also there is some evidence that bottlefeeding women feel themselves to be second class citizens in the maternity hospital (Kitzinger, 1979).

Perhaps it is not surprising that some mothers felt uncertain and anxious about feeding the baby, and the lower scores for young and primiparous women confirm this. However, it is obvious that many of them gained confidence as the days and weeks went on, due no doubt to the support from midwives, family and friends.

Midwives recognition of distress about feeding

The interviews held with the hospital midwives identified 54 women who were distressed about feeding their babies, and the community midwives also identified mothers who were distressed when they arrived home from the hospital. However it must be pointed out that these were not all the 54 women who later scored low emotional well-being. The link with emotional well-being and midwives recognition of feeding distress is significant (p=0.003) but it operates primarily through the link with the self-image in feeding factor (p=0.0001). This recognition by the midwives is important for several reasons; it confirms that the mother's self-image in feeding score really reflected how she was coping in the early postnatal days, it indicates that midwives have a high degree of skill in identifying vulnerable women at a very early stage, and from the comments written by the mothers it is obvious that many midwives provided very helpful and encouraging advice and encouragement. The picture which is conjured up is one in which some vulnerable women found themselves locked into a spiral of demoralization while others were given the help they needed to overcome it.

The nature of the help which these mother's need described much more effectively by Flint (1986), and Currell (1990) in her description of focused care, which is not so much problem solving as listening and honouring how women feel. It may have been the lack of focused care which made the following factors so detrimental to the mother's well-being.

Self-image in feeding, conflicting advice and lack of sleep in hospital

There is no doubt that conflicting advice had an eroding effect upon self-image in feeding and this was exacerbated by sleep disturbance in hospital.

Conflicting advice

Women who complained of conflicting advice had much lower scores for self-image in feeding six weeks later. Their numbers were large, almost 40 per cent complained. Conflicting advice has reared its ugly head in almost every study of maternal satisfaction with midwifery care (Williams, 1988; Thomson, 1989; Porter and McIntyre, 1989; Murphy-Black, 1994). Its causes are many:

- fragmentation of care among many different staff, including doctors and health visitors;
- telling women what to do rather than listening to how she feels;
- countermanding the advice of colleagues, confusing the mothers and reducing some of them to tears!

Not every woman is as strong as the one who commented:

> "I had so much conflicting advice from different midwives that in the end I told them to sod off and got on with it myself."

The emphasis is on conflicting advice rather than different advice, and this distinction holds a clue for the way that advice is delivered. If midwives and other staff started by enquiring what had already been advised and then built upon it, explaining why a new approach might be useful, then a good deal of frustration and distress could be avoided.

Perhaps the real answer to the problem of conflicting advice is two-fold. Midwives, doctors and health visitors need to be a lot more gracious of their colleagues advice and not contradict it unless it was absolutely essential. All staff need to learn the art of being encouraging and praising when seeking to support women who are embarking on this vital task which so enhances and enriches maternal-child relationships.

Lack of sleep in hospital

Lack of sleep in hospital affected self-image in feeding (p=0.01) and is significantly related to the emotional well-being score (p=0.01). It was not related to trait anxiety or satisfaction with motherhood (see Table 6.9). The effects of sleep disturbance on women may not always be recognized by midwives because disturbance of sleep is so much a part of the task of caring for a baby. Crying babies, though, are not the only cause of sleep disturbance, although inflexible rooming-in patterns in two hospitals made that situation much worse than it need have been.

It is easy for staff to forget how difficult it is to sleep in hospital. Hospitals are busy, noisy places. But the day-time is also busy and there was evidence from the mothers comments and later observation of postnatal wards that many women who have been in labour during the night were disturbed by ward routines when sleeping the following day. Several women spoke of being unable to sleep during the day following delivery and then being left exhausted, but expected to care for her baby the following night. In the observation of wards which formed part of the study, a record of the need for sleep was rarely seen in the mother's care records.

Increasing opportunities for rest

Part of the solution to this problem lies in arranging for mothers to go home as soon as possible after the birth where they will be disturbed only by their own baby and where they may be able to get extra rest in the daytime. Another is to make sure that women who had a sleepless night, either in labour, caring for a fretful baby, or in pain from stitches, recovering from caesarean section, for instance, are enabled to sleep undisturbed and for as long as possible, the following day.

There needs to be a fundamental change in the way wards are run, and in the attitudes of all types of staff and visitors, that the mother's sleep is vital if she is to recover from the effort of labour and the work of caring for her baby. Further research (Ball and Stanley, 1984) explored ways of increasing and improving the sleep of mothers. Rest periods when the ward is closed have been shown to be beneficial, single rooms should be kept for the use of mothers who have had a bad night with the baby, or have been in labour during the night, and mothers should be supplied with "Do not disturb" notices which they can hang up when they wish. Above all, the following edict based on a later survey of activities in postnatal wards should become part of the ethos, training and discipline of all staff working in postnatal care;

> **It should be regarded as a cardinal sin ever to wake a sleeping mother ... and this applies to medical staff of all grades, but especially junior doctors "doing rounds", midwives however senior, cleaners who pull the beds out to clean behind them because "this is their day for doing it", mother's visitors, newspaper sellers, etc.**

Satisfaction with motherhood

Almost all the women in the sample had high levels of satisfaction with motherhood and apart from the three who scored low satisfaction, there were no significant differences in the range of scores in relation to parity (p=0.4181) social class (p=0.5638), age (p=0.5057), breast or bottlefeeding (0.30059), type of labour (p=0.1360) or delivery (p=0.1307). The 33 women who had been separated from their own mothers before the age of eleven (Frommer and O'Shea, 1973) were just as satisfied with motherhood as those who had not (p=-0.7869).

Mothers with low self-image in feeding scores were no less satisfied than the others (p=0.1707), neither were those who complained of lack of sleep in hospital (p=0.1192).

In terms of midwifery practice and of understanding something more of the processes surrounding maternal-infant attachment, the most important and statistically significant factors related to satisfaction with motherhood were the mother's birth feelings, and whether or not she fed her baby in the delivery suite.

Birth feelings

It is not easy to provide any explanation for these feelings, nor indeed should they need explaining. How a woman feels immediately after the birth of her baby is made up of many things, the experience of labour, her degree of exhaustion, her original feelings about whether or not the pregnancy was wanted.

These are reflected in some other data: women who said they were "looking forward to being a mother" rather than "getting it over" were more likely to express themselves as "gloriously happy" after the birth (p=0.0035). Other factors, however, did not make a difference; parity (p=0.4921), age (p=0.1407), type of feeding (p=0.0607), although breastfeeders had slightly higher scores. The type of labour (p=0.2717) and delivery (p=0.7397) made no difference, but the mother's expectation of labour had a bearing on her feelings, with those who felt that the labour had been worse than expected much more inclined to express their birth feelings as being "too tired to care" (p=0.001). However, this was not the case with the pain score, mothers who said the pain was bad or unbearable most of the time did not have any less positive birth feelings than those who had not been distressed by the pain (p=0.1705).

Feeding the baby in the delivery suite

In view of the many factors listed above which did not impact upon the mother's birth feelings, the fact that those who fed their baby in the delivery suite scored significantly more positive birth feelings (p=0.0228) gives us an important clue for enhancing satisfaction with motherhood and thereby increasing emotional well-being. In view of the work of Klaus and Kennel *et al* (1975, 1982) perhaps we should not be surprised. What is of concern, however, is that the enabling of mothers to give feeds seems to be arbitrary and subject to attitudes of staff or pressure of work in the delivery suite, and that the importance of this first hour for the baby and its parents, and for the establishment of breastfeeding was not given recognition in the way the delivery suites were run. It was also notable that women who had their husband, partner, mother or some other friend with them during labour and delivery scored more positive birth feelings and this result just reached significance level (p=0.0515). The recent work on the effect of the presence of 'doulas' (Klaus *et al*, 1986) adds significance to this relationship. Also it may be that midwives were more likely to delay the moving of a mother to postnatal care if her husband or some other helper was with her.

There is no doubt that the mothers who did feed their babies within the first hour were breastfeeders (p=0.0001), over 20 years of age (p=0.01) and from social class I, II and III n/manual (p=0.01). The type of labour or delivery was not significant (see Tables 6.19, 6.20 in previous chapter) but women who had received Pethidine during labour were less likely to feed their baby (p=0.0001).

However not all the women who intended to breastfeed were given the opportunity, Table 6.20 in Chapter 6 shows that only 58 per cent of them suckled their babies in spite of hospital policies which advocated this. Bottlefeeding women fared even worse, in spite of the fact that the giving and receiving of a feed gives pleasure and that the "en-face" position can be achieved via bottlefeeding as well as by breastfeeding.

It is unlikely that it was the actual giving of a feed which made the difference, but that midwives and other staff gave the mother and her partner time together. The giving of a feed, almost entirely restricted to breastfeeders, "gave permission" for the parent to have time and space to delight in their baby and each other. This is so sad, after all, the birth follows 40 weeks of pregnancy and antenatal care designed to promote the health of the mother, baby and family. How dare we allow the business or routines of a delivery suite to interfere with these precious first moments.

The author believes that the solution lies in recognizing that there are **four** significant and important stages of labour which should become part of the training of all midwives and doctors.

The 'fourth stage' of labour - enhancing satisfaction with motherhood

The results of the study showed that maternal satisfaction with motherhood acted as a boost to emotional well-being, and that it was enhanced by close contact between the mother and her baby during the first hour after delivery. For many of the women in the study this close contact was made possible because they breastfed their baby whilst they were still in the labour ward.

Most midwifery and obstetric text-books recognize three stages of labour: the first stage of dilation of the cervix, leading to the second expulsive stage which results in the birth of the baby, followed by the third stage of expulsion of the placenta and contraction of the uterus to control haemorrhage. It is high time that a fourth stage of labour was recognized and became as important a part of the conduct of labour as the first three. This fourth stage is the time immediately following the birth when the mother and her newborn baby can come into close physical and emotional contact with each other. Although the work of Leboyer (1975), Klaus and Kennell (1982) and many others has stressed the importance of this contact, it still tends to be regarded as an optional extra which may be possible if circumstances are favourable.

Birth is preceded by 40 weeks of pregnancy, during which time the maternity services have taken great care to ensure the birth of a healthy baby to a healthy mother. It is perhaps indicative of the foreshortened view of midwives and doctors that birth is seen as the climax of care, and that although sharing the moment of birth with the parents is enjoyed, the bustle of clearing up after a delivery, writing up the records and arranging a postnatal bed tends to distract from the importance of enabling the parents and baby to spend an uninterrupted time together for as long as they wish.

The birth of their child is a peak experience in the life of its parents; it is a deeply emotional and personal moment which cannot be recaptured. When it is over the parents will separate for a time, the mother and baby going to the postnatal ward, and the father going home to spread the news to the rest of the family. Those who care for women during labour and childbirth should ensure that this period of time is regarded as sacrosanct and that nothing apart from immediate danger to the life of the mother or baby is allowed to disturb it. It is particularly important for the father of the baby, and his needs tend to be forgotten. He may not have an opportunity to be in such close contact with his infant for several days, and he may be going home exhausted but hopefully exhilarated by the experience he has just shared.

If the father of the baby is not with the mother during or immediately after the birth, she still needs to enjoy sharing this moment with some other companion or with the midwife or doctor who has cared for her during labour. The important thing is that she should be able to delight in her baby and to share that delight with someone else. She should also be praised for her achievement in giving birth; nothing saps joy or self-confidence more than an attitude which conveys that having a baby is a common occurrence and not particularly special!

The satisfactory completion of this stage of labour should therefore be regarded as requiring the same degree of attention and care as the first three stages, and no doctor or midwife should consider that his or her responsibilities are at an end until it has been fulfilled.

This fourth stage of labour will still need to be fulfilled even when it is not possible immediately after the birth either because the mother is anaesthetized or because the baby requires urgent attention or is stillborn. In the first instance a time of sharing between the baby's parents can be arranged as soon as the mother is able to enter into it fully, and the same pattern of uninterrupted time should be followed. If the baby is ill, the mother must be enabled to see and touch him before he is whisked away to special care. She and her partner may then need a time to comfort each other. When a stillbirth occurs, many parents find it helpful to see and touch the baby, delighting and grieving in his unfulfilled beauty and potential. This opportunity for parents to grieve together over a dead or sick baby is just as important as the time spent rejoicing over a healthy child, and nothing should be allowed to interfere with it (White et *al*, 1984; Murray and Callan, 1988).

Midwives have a particular role to play in ensuring that this fourth stage is fulfilled for all parents. Midwives are the key people in determining the way that delivery suites are run. It is the midwives who take responsibility for the conduct of the majority of births in this country, and where the labour does not result in a normal delivery, it is the midwife who takes over the care of the mother from the doctor and who organizes the transfer to the postnatal ward. Midwives therefore have a particular responsibility to ensure that the fostering of healthy parent-child relationships becomes an integral part of the care given, and that junior medical staff and medical and midwifery students are instructed in its significance.

Conclusion

The results of the study identified how complex, intricate and personal are reactions to motherhood. There is no "proper" or "correct" way to adjust to this demanding and delightful experience, neither is there any "proper" or "normal" time within which mothers and babies "ought" to be coping well. Rather, it has highlighted the importance of focusing attention on the needs of individual women, praising their prowess in giving birth and nurturing their babies, and enabling them to proceed at their own pace in assuming all the responsibilities for the care of their babies.

The study has shown how patterns and events of postnatal care, which begin with the birth of the baby can have a beneficial or detrimental effect upon the mother's reactions and via her reactions upon the welfare of her baby and her family. Midwives, doctors and all other staff who are privileged to share in the care and experiences of parents at the birth of children have a great responsibility to enhance and enrich the experience, and this is particularly important when the mother is vulnerable to distress because of predisposing factors and events over which she has little or no control. Providing focused, individual care for as long as it is needed is the key to reducing distress, identifying the danger of depression and enriching the experience for women and those who attend them.

CHAPTER 8

Reactions to Motherhood: The Role of Postnatal Care

Childbirth and motherhood should be a time of fulfilment and joy for both mothers, fathers, siblings and the extended family, and the appropriateness of the care which surrounds and underpins motherhood should be a matter of concern to the whole of society.

The aims of postnatal care

The purpose of all maternity care is to enable a woman to be successful in becoming a mother, giving birth to a healthy infant and embarking in strength and confidence upon her lifelong commitment of motherhood. The objectives of maternity care must, therefore, be as concerned with the emotional and psychological processes as they are with the physiological.

The latter half of the 20th century has seen dramatic changes in the provision of skilled care for women during pregnancy, labour and childbirth. In the United Kingdom the establishment and development of the National Health Service, the improvement of the general health of the population, the growth of obstetric and paediatric knowledge and technology, the emergence of midwifery research have all served to reduce the levels of maternal and neonatal mortality and morbidity to a degree undreamt of by the early pioneers of maternity care.

However, although major changes have taken place in the way that maternity care is organized, and in the policies of delivery suites and neonatal units, comparatively little attention has been paid to postnatal care, which tends to be given a lower status after the dramas and excitement of labour and delivery. Yet it is during this time that all the mother's pent-up mixture of feelings are released: fear of labour, joy at a healthy baby, uncertainty about being able to cope with the baby and all his or her needs. No doubt, these are some of the elements which underlie the common phenomenon of the 'third day blues'.

The majority of mothers will make a happy and confident adjustment to motherhood, some may take a little longer than others, some will need more help than others and sadly some will become depressed. An unhappy woman will not be able fully to enter into this life-enhancing situation. She may feel that she is failing her husband and baby, she may feel afraid and trapped in a situation she can't manage. It is during this time that midwives in particular have such an opportunity to influence the situation.

The art of postnatal care lies in understanding how a mother is coping, how she feels about herself and her baby, acknowledging the validity of those feelings and tailoring the pattern and degree of care to suit individual women's needs.

The objectives of postnatal care are three-fold.

1. Promoting the physical recovery from the effects of pregnancy, labour and delivery, of the mother and baby.
2. Establishing sound infant-feeding practices and fostering good maternal-child relationships.
3. Strengthening the mother's confidence in herself and in her ability to care for her baby in her own particular social, cultural and family situation.

Whilst all those involved in providing care for mothers and babies would agree with these objectives, some of the structures and processes of postnatal care which obtained at the time of the study and which largely still exist, make them difficult to achieve.

The main focus of postnatal care has traditionally been that of ensuring physical recovery of the mother from the rigours of pregnancy and labour, and establishing infant feeding patterns. The emotional and psychological needs of mothers have not received as much attention until recently and there has been an assumption that emotional and psychological needs will automatically be met if the first two aspects of care are satisfied. Much of the organization of postnatal care has been based on this premise.

However, the work of Lazarus (1966, 1969), Caplan (1969), Caplan and Killelia (1976), Klaus and Kennell (1982), Klaus et al (1986) and the growing understanding of factors associated with the high incidence of postnatal distress and depression (Cox 1982, Cox *et al*, 1986; Murray 1988; Holden et al, 1989) does not allow us to hold such a view. The results of this study have revealed how care factors can influence the pattern and pace of adjustment to motherhood.

Changes since the first edition

In the first edition of this book a number of processes were noted which frustrated continuity of care and also promoted a routine-based approach to postnatal care delivery. Some are still relevant and will be discussed shortly, but it must be pointed out that one of the many delights of revising this work has been to note how, in the eight years between the two editions, so much research has informed midwifery practice (Sleep *et al*, 1984; 1987; 1988a; 1988b; Kirkham ,1989; 1993; Laryea, 1984; 1989; Thomson, 1989) and many efforts have been made to improve continuity of care (Flint, 1991; Page, 1988; Currell, 1990).

Such developments have been mainly in the realm of care processes. Now in 1994 as a result of the Report of the Winterton Committee Report (House of Commons, 1992) and its uptake by the midwifery profession (Ball *et al*, 1992; Page, 1993) and the Department of Health (1993) major changes to the structures as well as the processes of care are beginning to take shape.

Structures and processes of postnatal care

Donabedian, who has pioneered the understanding and development of quality assurance in health services (Donabedian, 1966; 1980) argues that good health outcomes are the product of effective care processes, which in turn are rooted in appropriate health service structures. This concept is illustrated by the results of the study and some aspects of the structures and processes of the maternity service at the time of the study.

Difficulties arising from the hospital environment

The study highlighted a number of care issues whose roots lay in the culture of the hospital environment, and in the pressure of work created for midwives and doctors by this fragmented system of care.

In all the many changes in the maternity service over the years, the main one is that of making the hospital the normal place for childbirth. As a consequence, almost all babies are born in hospital, and this is likely to remain the norm, even though women now have more choice and some of the resistance to home deliveries has lessened.

While there has been numerous publications about hospital births (Chard and Richards, 1977; Kitzinger and Davis, 1978; Tew, 1990) little attention has been focused upon the subsequent postnatal care and the way it is organized.

For the majority of women postnatal care begins in the hospital delivery suite followed by a period of time in the postnatal ward where she may share a room with two, four, six or even 30 other mothers. Many women will prefer to go home as soon as possible after birth, others will either want or need to stay longer, either to recover from a difficult birth, or to become confident in feeding the baby, or to have a rest from a demanding home situation.

Over the years maternity hospitals have developed a number of policies on discharging mothers and babies, many of which do not readily fit the mother's expectations. Other factors in hospital-based care meant that mothers frequently meet with routine or task-centred, rather than individualized care.

In the community services, most had care policies which meant that midwives met women during pregnancy and then cared for them after the birth, thus having an opportunity to build up good relationships. However this was easier to arrange in some areas rather than in others. Where a hospital provided a service for mothers from many different geographical areas (as was the case with hospital 3 in the study) or where midwives were not attached to sympathetic general practitioner practices, this proved difficult to organize. More recent research (Murphy-Black, 1994) indicates that this is still a problem in some areas.

Intensity of work in maternity hospitals

One of the largely unrecognized effects of concentrating births within maternity hospitals has been the intensity of the work created. Dealing with this intensity creates organizational patterns which make it difficult to provide continuity of care or carer. The closure of small maternity units during the last two decades has meant that most maternity hospitals are providing care for large numbers of women, ranging from 3500 to 4500 births a year, and in the biggest units 6000+ births a year.

Maternity care is an entirely emergency-driven service, at least in terms of the major part of the work, intrapartum and postnatal care. Fluctuations in workload in delivery suites means that sometimes there are too many staff available and at others times too few. Although the development of workload measures based on clinical indicators (Ball, 1993) gives an overall measure of staffing requirements, it cannot predict the variability of workload on any particular day.

Postnatal wards are also very busy places. Women are admitted at any time during the day or night after giving birth, and the majority stay for 48 hours before going home to the care of the community midwife. This means that the population of a ward is constantly changing. It also means that mother's go home at just about the time that babies are beginning to show more interest in breastfeeding and breasts are becoming very full.

Rituals

Another strange anomaly existed at the time of the study and still does in many hospitals. This was the concept of the 'first day' after birth. Somewhere in the mists of midwifery administration, certainly stretching beyond the author's first acquaintance with maternity care 40 years ago, it was decided that postnatal 'days' should be recognized according to whether or not a baby was born between midnight and noon, or noon and midnight. If a baby was born at 11.30 hours on, for example, a Monday, then that day was counted as the first postnatal day, and if the mother had planned to go home on the second day post-delivery she would leave on the next day. But if the baby was foolish enough to arrive at 12.30 hours on the same Monday, then this day would not count as the first postnatal day. Instead Tuesday would be considered to be the 'first' day and the mother and her baby would then leave on Wednesday, the official 'second' day. This meant that mothers who gave birth within an hour of each other, had different lengths of time in the ward, even though both had arranged to go home on the 'second' postnatal day. This pattern was rigidly adhered to by both midwives and junior doctors but the mothers failed to understand it and it was the cause of numerous complaints. This strange situation serves to illustrate the way in which rituals develop which have no logical basis.

Routines

As the pace of life in postnatal wards is so fast, a system of giving care evolved which was based upon having set times for carrying out certain tasks, to ensure that they were all done. In the wards observed in the study, this led to various 'rounds' during the day in which the same aspect of care was undertaken for all mothers, temperature rounds, examination of breast and involution of uterus, checking on feeding etc. During the day junior doctors also did rounds, followed in many hospitals by a phlebotomist or a physiotherapist each with their quota of mothers to be seen. This was one of the major causes of disturbance of rest in the wards, and created an environment where conflicting advice could flourish.

All of these activities produce a routine or task-centred approach in which the woman as an individual is swamped and her care may be fragmented. It also produced an unsatisfactory climate of care in which the midwives felt equally frustrated!

Staff changes

A further issue in the hospital environment is the frequent changeover of staff. At regular intervals, student and staff midwives rotate from day to night duty and to different parts of the service. So do medical students, and junior doctors who generally change every six months or so. This makes not only for a fluctuating set of people engaged in postnatal care, but also a variation in the level of personal and professional skills.

Shift working

Organizing care in hospital inevitably leads to the need for duty rosters, designed to ensure that adequate qualified staff are available 24 hours a day. Working on different shifts, made it difficult for one midwife to see through the care of any particular woman.

These situations all tend to encourage the adoption and retention of routine-centred patterns of care because such patterns help to ensure that vital aspects of care are not neglected and help inexperienced staff to cope with the intensive demands of postnatal wards.

At the time of the study there was very little development of the principle of primary or team nursing. It must be said, however, that in spite of these difficulties, hospital midwives made great efforts to give personal care, and that since then, tremendous efforts have been made to improve the situation particularly through the use of teams of midwives working either in association with a particular consultant or area of a hospital, and in the growth of midwifery managed delivery suites (Department of Health, 1993; Morris-Thompson, 1993). In these ways, the number of staff involved with each mother is reduced, thus increasing the opportunity for developing relationships and providing increased continuity of care during the relatively short time in hospital.

Proposed changes in the structure and processes of maternity care

Many of the issues described above formed a substantial part of the evidence submitted to the Winterton Committee (House of Commons, 1992). One of the main thrusts of its conclusions and recommendations was that of recognizing that the existing structures of the service needed to be changed to enable more personalized care to be provided to women. It was argued that the main vehicle through which such changes could be made lay in the freeing of midwives from attachment to wards, departments and doctors in order to 'staff the women' - giving care to mothers throughout the pregnancy, supporting them through labour and delivery wherever it took place, and then providing the postnatal care.

The broad principles are summarized below in an extract from the list of eight recommendations (House of Commons, 1992, p. ixxx).

> the relationship between the mother and her care-giver is recognized as being of fundamental importance

> schemes should be set up which enable women to get to know one or two health professionals during pregnancy who will be with them during labour and delivery ... and will continue the care of mother and baby after the birth

> the majority of maternity care should be community based ...

> the woman having a baby should be seen as the focus of care, and that professionals providing that care should develop arrangements ... to ensure full and equal cooperation with all those charged with her care

These recommendations laid emphasis on the processes of care which were to be achieved. In their recommendations regarding the work of midwives, changes in the structure of maternity care were proposed, and these are summarized below.

We recommend that:

> the status of midwives as professionals is acknowledged in their terms and conditions of employment

> that we should move as rapidly as possible towards a situation in which midwives have their own caseload and take full responsibility for the women under their care

> the midwives be given the opportunity to establish and run midwifery managed maternity units within and outside hospitals

> that the right of midwives to admit women to NHS hospitals should be made explicit

> (Extracts from House of Commons, 1992, p. ixxii)

These proposals present an opportunity to change maternity care both in hospital and community. Further discussion of their implications and plans for their achievement have followed (Ball *et al*, 1992; Expert Committee on Maternity Care, Department of Health, 1993, South East Thames Regional Health Authority, 1992). Pilot schemes are already in action (One for One service; Centre for Midwifery Practice at Hammersmith and Queen Charlotte Special Health Authority and the launch of midwifery group practice in the South East Thames Regional Health Authority (1994). Both of these pilot systems will be the subject of research based evaluation. It is envisaged that groups of six midwives will care for 200+ women per annum and provide postnatal care to a limited number of other women whose care will primarily be provided by the obstetrician (Ball et *al*, 1992). Midwives working in caseload-based practices will be able to build relationships in pregnancy with the whole family, and to accompany the mother in labour, undertake the delivery, or if necessary stay with the mother who needs some emergency intervention during labour. Other midwives based primarily but not exclusively in hospital will provide focused care for women booked under the care of the obstetrician.

The changes now influencing the provision of midwifery services provide a glorious opportunity for 'loading the dice' in favour of good emotional outcomes. The onus on the midwifery profession is large, but its history and the enthusiastic commitment of present day midwives suggests that it will be able to meet the challenge.

It is to the midwives who will develop these structures and to the mother's whose expectations and experiences will shape them that this book is dedicated.

> For this reason I kneel before the Father from whom the whole family on earth and in heaven derives its name. I pray that out of His glorious riches He will strength you with power through His Spirit in your inner being. (Letter of Paul to the Ephesians, Ch. 3, v. 14-16.)

References

Affonso, D.D. (1984). 'Postpartum depression'. In: Field, P.A. (Ed). *Recent Advances in Nursing Series*. Edinburgh:Churchill Livingstone.

Arnold, M. (1960). *Emotion and Personality*. New York:Coumbia University Press.

Arizmendi, T.G., Affonso, D.D.(1984). 'Research on psychosocial factors and postnatal depression: a critique.' *Birth*, Vol. 11, Winter, pp. 237-40.

Bacon, C.J., Wylie, J.M. (1976). 'Mother's attitudes in infant feeding at Newcastle General Hospital in 1975'. British Medical Journal, i, pp.308-30.

Ball, J.A. (1981). 'The effects of the present patterns of maternity care upon the emotional needs of mothers: I, II and III.' *Midwives Chronicle*, 95, (1120), 150-54; (1121), 198-202; (1122), 231-33.

Ball, J.A. (1984). 'What happens now?' (RCM Supplement). *Nursing Times*, 80 (29), 3-5.

Ball, J.A. (1993). 'Workload measures in midwifery care.' In: Alexander, J., Levy, V., Roch, S. (Eds). *Further Advances in Midwifery - A Research-based Aproach*. Andover:Macmillan Press.

Ball, J.A., Flint, C., Garner, M., Jackson-Baker, A., Page, L. (1992). 'Who's Left Holding the Baby? Making the Most of Midwifery Resources'. Nuffield Institute for Health Services Studies. Leeds University, 71-75 Clarendon Road, Leeds, LS2 9PL.

Ball, J.A., Stanley, J. (1984). 'Stress and the mother'. (Supplement: RCM Professional Day Papers.) *Midwives Chronicle*, 97 (1162), xviii-xxii.

Beck, A.T., Ward, C.H., Mendelson, M., Mock, J., Erbaugh, J. (1961). 'An inventory for measuring depression.' *Archives of General Psychiatry*, 4, 561-71.

Beech, B.L. (1987). *Who's Having your Baby? A Health Rights Handbook for Maternity Care*. London: Camden Press.

Bernal, J. (1972). 'Crying during the first ten days of life and maternal response.' *Developmental Medicine and Child Neurology*, 4, 362-72.

Bowlby, J. (1951). *Maternal Care and Mental Health*. Bulletin of the World Health Organisation. London:HMSO.

Bowlby, J. (1961). 'Separation anxiety: a critical review of the literature'. *Journal of Child Psychology*, 15, 9-52.

Boyd, C., Sellers, L. (1982). *The British Way of Birth*. London:Pan Books.

British Medical Journal (1977). 'Helping mothers to love their babies.' *British Medical Journal*, September, 595-96.

Brockington, I.F., Cox-Roper, A. (1988). 'The nosology of puerperal mental illness.' In: Kumar, R., Brockington, I.F. (Eds). *Motherhood and Mental Illness*.

Broussard, E.R., Hartner, M.S.S. (1971). 'Further considerations regarding maternal perception of the newborn'. In: Jerome, J. (Ed). *Exceptional Infant: Studies in Abnormality*. Vol. 2, pp. 432-49. New York:Brunner-Mazel.

Brown, G., Harris, T. (1978). *Social Origins of Depression: A Study of Psychiatric Disorder in Women*. London:Tavistock.

Brown, W.A. (1979). *Psychological Care during Pregnancy and the Post-natal Period*. New York:Raven Press.

Campbell, A.V. (1984). Moderated Love: A Theology of Professional Care. London:SPCK.

Caplan, G. (1964). *Principles of Preventative Psychiatry*. London:Tavistock.

Caplan, G. (1969). *An Approach to Community Mental Health*. London:Tavistock.

Caplan, G., Killilea, M. (1976). *Support Systems and Mutual Help*. Orlando:Grune and Stratton.

Cattell, R.B., Scheier, I.H. (1961). *Meaning and Measurement of Neuroticism and Anxiety*. New York:Ronald Press.

Chalmers, I. (1978). 'Implications of the current debate on obstetric practice.' In: Kitzinger, S., Davis, J. (Eds). London:Oxford University Press.

Chalmers, I., Enkin, M., Keirse, M.J.N.C. (1989). *Effective Care in Pregnancy and Childbirth*. Oxford:Oxford University Press.

Chard, T., Richards, M. (Eds). (1977). 'Lessons for the future.' In: *Benefits and Hazards of the New Obstetrics*, pp. 157-63. London:Heinemann Medical Books.

Chertok, L. (1969). *Motherhood and Personality*. London:Tavistock.

Clayton, S. (1979). *Maternity Care: Some Patient's Views*. Newcastle Community Health Council Survey Report. Newcastle:NCHC.

Cogill, S., Caplan, H.L., Alexandra, H., Mordecai Robson, K., Kumar, R. (1986). 'Impact of maternal postnatal depression on cognitive development of young children'. *British Medical Journal*, 292, pp. 1165-67.

Cooper, P.J., Campbell, E.A., Day, A., Kennerley, H., Bond, A. (1988). 'Non-psychotic psychiatric disorder after childbirth: a prospective study of prevalence, incidence, course and nature.' *British Journal of Psychiatry*, 152, pp. 799-806.

Cox, B.S. (1974). 'Rooming in.' *Nursing Times*, 70, 1246-47.

Cox, J.L. (1978). 'Some socio-cultural determinants of psychiatric morbidity associated with childbearing.' In: Sandler, M. (Ed). *Mental Illness in Pregnancy and the Puerperium*, pp. 91-98. London:Oxford University Press.

Cox, J.L. (1983). 'Postnatal depression: A comparison of Scottish and African women'. *Social Psychiatry*, 18, pp. 25-28.

Cox, J.L. (1985). Paper given at a joint conference of the Marcé Society and the Royal College of Midwives, Kings Fund Centre, London, 8 March 1985.

Cox, J.L. (1986). *Postnatal Depression: A Guide for Health Professionals*. Edinburgh:Churchill Livingstone.

Cox, J.L. (1988). 'The life event of childbirth: sociocultural aspects of postnatal depression'. In: Kumar, R. and Brockington, I.F. (Eds). *Motherhood and Mental Illness*. London: Wright, Butterworth & Co. Ltd.

Cox, J.L. (1989). 'Can postnatal depression be prevented?' *Midwife, Health Visitor and Community Nurse,* 25, pp. 326-32.

Cox, J.L., Connor, Y., Kendell, R.E. (1982). 'Prospective study of the psychiatric disorders of childbirth'. *British Journal of Psychiatry,* 140, pp. 111-17.

Cox, J.L., Holden, J.M., Sagovsky, R. (1987). 'Detection of postnatal depression: development of the 10-item Edinburgh Postnatal Depression Scale'. *British Journal of Psychiatry,* 150, pp. 782-86.

Cox, J.L., Murray, D., Chapman, G. (1993). 'A controlled study of the onset, duration and prevalence of postnatal depression'. *British Journal of Psychiatry,* 163, pp. 27-31.

Currell, R. (1990). 'The organisation of midwifery care'. In: Alexander, J., Levy, V. and Roch, S. (Eds). *Antenatal Care: A Research-based Approach.* London:MacMillan Education.

Dalton, K. (1980). *Depression after Childbirth.* London:Oxford University Press.

Department of Health (1993). *Changing Childbirth.* The Report of the Expert Maternity Group. London: HMSO. .

Derlega, V.J., Janda, L.H. (1978). *Personal Adjustment: The Psychology of Everyday Life.* Glenview, Illinois:General Learning Press (subsidiary of Scott, Foresman and Co.).

DeVries, R.G. (1989). 'Care givers in pregnancy and childbirth'. In: Chalmers, I., Enkin, M. and Keirse, M.J.N.C. (Eds). *Effective Care in Pregnancy and Childbirth.* Oxford:Oxford University Press..

Donabedian, A. (1966). 'Evaluating the quality of medical care'. *Millband Memorial Quarterly,* 64, 3, pp. 66-206.

Donabedian, A. (1980). 'The definition of quality assurance and approaches to its measurement. AnnArbor, Health Administration Press.

Draramraj, C., Siac, G., Kierney, C.M., Harper, R.C., Pareck, A., Weissman, B. (1981). 'Observations on maternal preference for rooming-in Harper facilities.' *Paediatrics,* 67(5), 638-40.

Dunn, J.B., Richard, M.P.H. (1977). 'Observation of the developing relationship between the mother and baby in the neonatal period'. In: Schaffer, H.R. (Ed) *Studies in Mother-Infant Interaction,* pp. 427-53. London:Academic Press.

Elliott, S.A., Rugg, A.J., Watson, J.P., Brough, D.I. (1983). 'Mood changes during pregnancy and after the birth of a child'. *British Journal of Clinical Psychology,* 22, pp. 295-308.

Erikson, E.H. (1963). *Childhood and Society,* 2nd edn. New York:Norton.

Evans, F. (1988). 'Partnership to tackle poverty', Community Care, 792, pp.iv-vi.

Eysenck, H.J. (1959). *Manual of the Maudesley Personality Inventory.* London:University of London Press.

Eysenck, H.J., Eysenck, S.B.G. (1968). *Manual of the Eysenck Personality Questionnaire.* London:Hodder and Stoughton Educational Division.

Eysenck, H.J., Soueif, M.I., White, P.O. (1969). 'A joint factoral study of Guildford, Cattell and Eysenck scales.' In: Eysenck, H.J., Eysenck, S.B.G. (Eds). *Personality Structure and Measurement,* pp. 171-93. London:Routledge and Kegan Paul.

Filshie, S., Williams, J., Osbourn, M., Senior, O.E., Symonds, E.M., Backett, E.M. (1981). 'Post-natal care in hospital: time for a change.' *International Journal of Nursing Studies,* 18(2), 89-95.

Flint, C. (1986). *Sensitive Midwifery.* Oxford:Heinemann Medical Books.

Flint, C. (1991). 'Continuity of care provided by a group of midwives - the Know Your Midwife Scheme'. In: Robinson, S. and Thomson, A.M. (Eds). *Midwives, Research and Childbirth.* Vol. 2. London:Chapman and Hall.

Flint, C., Poulengeris, P. (1987). 'The "Know Your Midwife" report'. Available from: 49 Peckarmans Wood, Sydenham Hill, London SE26 6RZ.

Freud, S. (1940). *The Outline of Psychoanalysis.* London:Hogarth Press.

Frommer, E.A., O'Shea, G. (1973). 'Antenatal identification of women liable to have problems in managing their infants.' *British Journal of Psychiatry,* 123, 149-56.

Goldberg, D.P., Cooper, B., Eastwood, M.R., Kedward, H.B., Shepherd, M. (1974). 'A standardized psychiatric interview for use in community surveys.' *British Journal of Preventative and Social Medicine,* 24, 18-23.

Gruis, M. (1977). 'Beyond maternity: Post-partum concerns of mothers'. *American Journal of Maternal-Child Nursing,* 2 (3), pp. 182-88.

Hales, D.J., Lozoff, B., Sosa, R., Kennell, J.H. (1977). 'Defining the limits of the maternal sensitive period.' *Developmental Medicine and Child Neurology,* 19, 454.

Handley, S.L., Dunn, T.L., Baker, J.M. Cockshott, C., Gould, S. (1977). 'Mood changes in puerperium and plasma tryptophan and cortisol concentration'. *British Medical Journal,* 2, 18-22.

Handley, S.L., Dunn, T.L., Waldron, G., Baker, J. (1980). 'Trytophan, cortisol and puerperal mood'. *British*

Journal of Psychiatry, 136, pp. 490-505.

Hilgard, E.R., Atkinson, R.L., Atkinson, R.C. (1979). *Introduction to Psychology*, 7th edn. New York:Harcourt, Brace Jovanovich.

Hayward, J. (1975). Information: A Prescription against Pain. London:Royal College of Nursing.

Holden, J.M., Sagovsky, R., Cox, J.L. (1989). 'Counselling in a general practice setting: controlled study of health visitors intervention in treatment of postnatal depression'. *British Medical Journal*, 298, pp. 223-26.

Holmes, T.H., Rahe, R.H. (1967). 'Social readjustment rating scale'. *Journal of Psychosomoatic Research*, 11, 219.

Houldsworth, A. (1988). *Out of the Doll's House: The Story of Women in the Twentieth Century*. London:BBC Books.

House of Commons (1970). Domiciliary Midwifery and Maternity Bed Needs. Report of the Sub-Committee, Central Health Services Council, Standing Maternity and Midwifery Advisory Committee. London:HMSO.

House of Commons (1980). *Perinatal and Neonatal Mortality: Second Report from the Parliamentary Social Services Committee 1979-1980*. London: HMSO.

House of Commons (1992). *Second Report of the Health Committee on Maternity Services (Winterton)*. London: HMSO.

Houston, M.J. (1981). 'Breastfeeding: Success or Failure?' *Journal of Advanced Nursing*, 6, pp.447-54.

Inch, S. (1989). *Birthrights: A Parent's Guide to Modern Childbirth*. Second Edition. Green print. London: Merlin Press.

Kennell, J.H., Chesler, D., Wolfe, H., Jerauld, R., McAlpine, W., Kreger, N.C., Steffa, M., Klaus, M.H. (1974). 'Maternal behaviour one year after early and extended post-partum contact'. *Developmental Medicine and Child Neurology*, 16, 172-79.

Kirkham, M. (1989). 'Midwives and information giving during labour'. In: Robinson, S. and Thomson, A.M. (Eds). *Midwives, Research and Childbirth*. Vol. 1. London: Chapman and Hall.

Kirkham, M. (1993). 'Communication in midwifery'. In: Robinson, S. and Thomson, A.M. (Eds). *Midwives, Research and Childbirth*. London: Chapman and Hall.

Kitzinger, S. (1978). *Women as Mothers*. Oxford:Martin Robertson.

Kitzinger, S. (1979). *The Good Birth Guide*. Glasgow: Fontana paperbacks/HarperCollins.

Kitzinger, S. (1983). *Women's Experience of Sex*. London:Dorling Kindersley.

Kitzinger, S. (1989). 'Childbirth and society'. In: Chalmers, I., Enkin, M. and Keirse, M.J.N.C. (Eds). *Effective Care in Pregnancy and Childbirth*. Oxford:Oxford University Press.

Kitzinger, S., Davis, J. (Eds) (1978). *Place of Birth*. Oxford:Oxford University Press.

Klaus, M.H., Kennell, J.H. (1970). 'Human maternal behaviour at first contact with her young'. *Pediatrics*, 46(2), 187-92.

Klaus, M.H., Jerauld, R., Kreger, N.C., McAlpine, W., Steffa, M., Kennell, J.H. (1972). 'Maternal attachment: importance of the first post-partum days.' *New England Journal of Medicine*, 286, 460-63.

Klaus, M.H., Trause, M.A., Kennell, J.H. (1975). 'Does human maternal behaviour after delivery show a characteristic pattern?' In: Porter, E., O'connor, M. (Eds). *Parent-Infant Interaction*. Ciba Foundation Symposium No. 33. Amsterdam:Associated Scientific Publishers.

Klaus, M.H., Kennell, J.H. (1976). *Maternal-Infant Bonding*. St Louis: C.V. Mosby.

Klaus, M.H., Kennell, J.H. (1982). *Parent-Infant Bonding*. St Louis:C.V. Mosby.

Klaus, M.H., Kennell, J.H., Robertson, E.E., Sosa, R. (1986). 'Effects of social support during parturition on maternal and infant morbidity'. *British Medical Journal*, 293, pp. 585-87.

Kumar, R., Robson, K. (1978). 'Neurotic disturbance during pregnancy and the puerperium.' In: Sandler, M. (Ed). *Mental Illness in Pregnancy and the Puerperium*, pp. 40-51. Oxford:Oxford University Press.

Kumar, R., Robson, K.M. (1984). 'A prospective study of emotional disorders in childbearing women'. *British Journal of Psychiatry*, 144, pp. 35-47.

Laryea, M. (1984). *Post-Natal Care: The Midwife's Role*. London:Churchill Livingstone.

Laryea, M. (1989). 'Midwives and mothers perceptions of motherhood'. In: Robinson, S. and Thomson, A.M. (Eds). *Midwives, Research and Childbirth*. London: Chapman and Hall.

Lazarus, R.S. (1966). *Psychological Stress and the Coping Process*. New York:McGraw Hill.

Lazarus, R.S. (1969). *Patterns of Adjustment and Human Effectiveness*. New York:McGraw Hill.

Leboyer, F. (1975). *Birth Without Violence*. Aldershot:Wildwood House.

Leiderman, P.H., Seashore, M.J. (1975). 'Mother-infant separation: some delayed consequences.' In: Porter, E., O'Connor, M. (Eds). *Parent-Infant Interaction*, pp. 213-39. Ciba Foundation Symposium No. 33. Amsterdam:Associated Scientific Publishers.

Lishman, A. (1972). 'Selective factors in memory. II. Affective disorders.' *Psychological Medicine*, 2, 248-53.

Llewellyn Davies, M. (1979). *Maternity: Letters from Working Women.* London:Virago.

Lynch, M.A., Roberts, J., Gordon, M. (1976). 'Child abuse: early warning in the maternity hospital.' *Developmental Medicine and Child Neurology,* 18, 759-66.

McClellan, M.S., Cabianca, W.A. (1980). 'Effects of early mother-infant contact following caesarean birth'. *Obstetrics and Gynaecology,* 56, 1, 52-55.

Maslow, A.H. (1970). *Motivation and Personality.* New York and London:Harper and Row.

Melluish, E.C., Gambles, C., Kumar, R. (1988). 'Maternal mental illness and the mother-infant relationship'. In: Kumar, R. and Brockington, I.F. (Eds). *Motherhood and Mental Illness.* London: Wright, Butterworth & Co. Ltd.

Methven, R. (1989). 'Recording an obstetric history or relating to a pregnant woman?' In: Robinson, S. and Thomson, A.M. (Eds). *Midwives, Research and Childbirth.* London: Chapman and Hall.

Morris-Thompson, P. (1993). 'A historical perspective on maternity services and the Leicester Royal Infirmary approach to the Winterton Report's recommendations'. *Journal of Nursing Management,* 1, pp. 31-37.

Murphy-Black, T. (1994). 'Care in the community during the postnatal period'. In: Robinson, S. and Thomson, A.M. (Eds). *Midwives, Research and Childbirth.* London: Chapman and Hall.

Murray, L. (1988). 'Effects of postnatal depression on infant development: direct studies of early mother-infant interactions'. In: Kumar, R. and Brockington, I.F. (Eds). *Motherhood and Mental Illness.* London: Wright, Butterworth & Co. Ltd.

Murray, J., Callan, V.J. (1988). 'Predicting adjustment to perinatal death'. *British Journal of Medical Psychology,* 61, pp. 237-44.

Newton, N. (1955). *Maternal Emotions.* New York:Harper and Row.

Nilsson, A. (1972). 'Parental emotional adjustment'. In: Morris, N. (Ed). *Psychosomatic Medicine in Obstetrics and Gynaecology.* New York:Wiley.

Niven, C. (1994). 'Coping with labour pain: the midwife's role'. In: Robinson, S. and Thomson, A.M. (Eds). *Midwives, Research and Childbirth.* Vol. 3. London: Chapman and Hall.

Nuckalls, C.B., Cassell, J., Kaplan, B.H. (1972). 'Psycho-social assets, life-crises and the prognosis of pregnancy'. *American Journal of Epidemiology,* 95, 431-34.

Oakley, A. (1980). *Women Confined.* Oxford:Martin Robertson.

Oakley, A. (1994). 'Giving support in pregnancy: the role of research midwives in a randomised controlled trial'. In: Robinson, S. and Thomson, A.M. (Eds). *Midwives, Research and Childbirth.* Vol. 3. London: Chapman and Hall.

Oates, M. (1984). 'Significance of moving house for women with post-natal depression'. (Personal Communication.)

O'Hara, M.W., Rehm, L.P., Campbell, S.B. (1982). 'Predicting depressive symptomatology. Cognitive behavioural models and postpartum depression'. *Journal of Abnormal Psychology,* 91, pp. 457-461.

O'Hara, M.W., Rehm, L.P., Campbell, S.B. (1983). 'Postpartum depression: a role for social network and life-stress variables'. *Journal of Nervous and Mental Disease,* 171, pp. 336-341.

O'Hara, M.W., Neunaber, D.J., Zekowski, E.M. (1984). 'A prospective study of postpartum depression: prevalence, course, and predictive factors.' *Journal of Abnormal Psychology,* 93, pp. 158-71.

O'Hara, M., Zekoski, E.M. (1988). 'Postpartum depression: a comprehensive review'. In: Kumar, R. and Brockington, I.F. (Eds). *Motherhood and Mental Illness.* London: Wright, Butterworth & Co. Ltd.

O'Hara, M.W., Neunaber, D.J., Zekoski, E.M. (1990). 'A prospective study of postpartum depression: prevalence, course and predictive factors'. *Journal of Abnormal Psychology,* 93, pp. 153-67.

Oppenheim, A.N. (1966). *Questionnaire Design and Attitude Measurement.* London:Heinemann.

Page, L. (1988). 'The midwife's role in modern health care'. In: Kitzinger, S. (Ed). *The Midwife Challenge.* London:Unwin Hyman/Pandora Press.

Page, L. (1993). 'Changing childbirth: a renewal of the maternity services'. *British Journal of Midwifery,* 1, 4, pp. ??-??.

Paykel, E.S., Emms, E.M., Fletcher, J., Rossaby, E.S. 'Life events and social support in puerperal depression'. *British Journal of Psychiatry,* 136, pp. 339-46.

Pitt, B. (1968). ' "Atypical" depression following childbirth'. *British Journal of Psychiatry,* 114, 1325-35.

Porter, M., McIntyre, S. (1989). 'Psychosocial effectiveness of antenatal and postnatal care'. In: Robinson, S. and Thomson, A.M. (Eds). *Midwives, Research and Childbirth.* London:Chapman and Hall.

Raskin, A., Schulterbrandt, J., Reatig, N., McKeon, J. (1970). 'Differential response to chlorpomazine, imipramine and placebo'. *Archives of General Psychiatry,* 23, pp. 164-73.

Reid, M., Garcia, J. (1989). 'Women's views of care during pregnancy and childbirth'. In: Chalmers, I., Enkin, M. and Keirse, M.J.N.C. (Eds). *Effective Care in Pregnancy and Childbirth.* Oxford: Oxford University Press.

Romito, P. (1989). 'Unhappiness after childbirth'. In: Chalmers, I., Enkin, M. and Keirse, M.J.N.C. (Eds).

Effective Care in Pregnancy and Childbirth. Oxford:Oxford University Press.

Rosen, B., Stein, M.J. (1980). 'Children and abusive women'. *American Journal of Diseases of Childhood,* 134, 946-51.

Seligman, M.E.P. (1975). *Helplessness: On Depression, Development and Death.* San Francisco: W.H.Freeman.

Shields, D. (1978). 'Nursing care in labour and patient satisfaction'. *Journal of Advances in Nursing,* 3(6), 535-50.

Siegel, E. (1982). 'Early and extended maternal-infant contact: a critical review'. *American Journal of Diseases of Childhood,* 136, March, pp. 251-57.

Sleep, J., Grant, A., Garcia, J., Elbourne, D., Spencer, J.A.D., Chalmers, I. (1984). 'West Berkshire perineal management trial'. *British Medical Journal,* 28, pp. 587-90.

Sleep, J., Grant, A. (1987). 'Pelvic floor exercises in post-natal care - the report of a randomised controlled trial to compare an intensive regimen with the programme in current use'. *Midwifery,* 3, pp. 158-64.

Sleep, J., Grant, A. (1988a). 'Routine use of salt of savlon bath concentrate during bathing in the immediate post-partum period - a randomised controlled trial'. *Nursing Times,* 84, (21), pp. 55-57.

Sleep, J., Grant, A. (1988b). 'The relief of perineal pain following childbirth: a survey of midwifery practice'. *Midwifery,* 4, pp. 118-22.

South East Thames Regional Health Authority (1992). *Maternity Services of the Future: Consensus Statement.* South East Thames Regional Health Authority, Thrift House, Collington Avenue, Bexhill-on-Sea, East Sussex, TN39 3NQ.

South East Thames Regional Health Authority (1994). *People for Health: Midwifery Group Practices 1994-1996.* South East Thames Regional Health Authority, Thrift House, Collington Avenue, Bexhill-on-Sea, East Sussex, TN39 3NQ.

Stein, A., Cooper, P.J., Campbell, E.A., Day, A., Altham, M.E. (1989). 'Social adversity and perinatal complications: their relation to postnatal depression'. *British Medical Journal,* 298, pp. 1073-74.

Stopher, P.R., Meyburg, A.H. (1979). *Survey Sampling and Multivariate Analysis for Social Scientists and Engineers.* Lexington, Mass., USA:Lexington Books, D.G. Heath & Co.

Tew, M. (1990). *Safer Childbirth? A Critical History of Maternity Care.* London:Chapman and Hall.

Thomson, A. (1989).'Why don't women breastfeed?' In: Robinson, S. and Thomson, A.M. (Eds). *Midwives, Research and Childbirth.* London: Chapman and Hall.

Tod, E.D.M. (1964). 'Puerperal depression: a prospective epidemiology study'. *Lancet,* II, 1264.

Watson, J.P., Elliott, S.A., Rugg, A.J., Brough, D.I. (1984). 'Psychiatric disorders in pregnancy and the first postnatal year'. *British Journal of Psychiatry,* 144, pp. 453-62.

Weinmann, J. (1981). *An Outline of Psychology as Applied to Medicine.* Bristol: John Wright.

Weiss, R.S. (1976). 'Transition states and other stressful situations: their nature and programs for their management.' In: Caplan, G., Killelia, M. (Eds) *Support Systems and Mutual Help,* pp. 211-32. New York:Grune and Stratton.

White, M.P., Reynolds, B., Evans, J.J. (1984). 'Handling of death in special care nurseries and parental grief'. *British Medical Journal,* 289, pp. 167-69.

Williams, S. (1988). Maternity survey. Ayrshire and Arran Health Board.

Wilson-Barnett, J. (1979). *Stress in Hospital: Patients' Psychological Reactions to Illness and Health Care.* Edinburgh:Churchill Livingstone.

Wilson-Barnett, J., Carrigy, A. (1978). 'Factors influencing patients' emotional reaction to hospitalization.' *Journal of Advanced Nursing,* 3(3), 221-29.

* Biblical references are taken from The Holy Bible; New International Version. London:Hodder & Stoughton.

Appendix I: Copies of Questionnaire, score sheets and Interview schedules used

RESEARCH STUDY: EMOTIONAL NEEDS OF MOTHERS

·Interview Schedule(1) Ante-Natal

	1	*2*	*3*
Unit No			

	4	*5*	*6*
Client No			

	7	*8*
Age		

Marital Status;   1. Married 2. Single 3.Seperated/divorced
> *9* □

Living with Partner?   1. Yes   2. No
> *10* □

Parity;   Primigravida. 1.Yes 2. No
> *11* □

No. of previous live births
> *12* □

No. of stillbirths/terminations
> *13* □

No. of infant deaths
> *14* □

Age of youngest child
> *15* *16* □□

Desired sex of infant; 1. Male 2. Female 3. Doesn't matter
> *17* □

Employment;   Husband employed at present? 1.Yes 2. No
Present or previous job
> *18* □

Client; 1. Maternity leave
2. Left work this pregnancy
3. Not employed before pregnancy
4. Other
> *19* □

Social class category
> *20* □

Early seperation from mothering figure?   1. Yes 2. No
> *21* □

Eysenck Scores;   E. Score
> *22* *23* □□

N. Score
> *24* *25* □□

E. Score; 1. High 2. Average 3. Low
> *26* □

N. Score; 1. High 2. Average 3. Low
> *27* □

What are you most looking forward to?
1."Getting it over" 2. Reaction of husband/children
3. Becoming a mother 4. Getting figure back
5. Going home with baby 6. Other
> *28 29 30* □□□
> *31 32 33* □□□

What if any, are your main anxie.ties/fears?
1. Not coping with labour/delivery 2. Pain
3. Care of older children
4. Ante-natal admission
5. Abnormal baby   6. Other
> *34 35 36* □□□
> *37 38 39* □□□

Any other comments

RESEARCH STUDY: EMOTIONAL NEEDS OF MOTHERS

Unit No | 0 | 0 | 4 |

Client No | | | |

Interview Schedule (2) Post-Labour

Date of delivery

Time of delivery (hours)   1. 0001–0600   2. 0601–1200
                            3. 1201–1800   4. 1801–2400

7 | |

Gestation at time of delivery (weeks)

8 9
| | |

LABOUR AND DELIVERY:

Labour;   1.Spontaneous   2. Induced 3. Active Management

10 | |

Length of labour (hours)

11 12
| | |

Pain relief   1. Epidural only   2. Epidural+sedation
                 3. Sedation+/–N O   4. N O only
                 5. Elective G.A.   6. No pain relief
                 7. Other

13 | |

Emergency G.A.   1. Yes   2. No

14 | |

Delivery   1. Normal   2. Forceps   3. Breech
                 4. Vacuum ext. 5.L.S.C.S. 6. Other

15 | |

Twin delivery   1. Yes 2. No

16 | |

Perineum   1. Tear   2. Episiotomy 3. Episiotomy+tear 4. Intact

17 | |

Third stage   1. Normal 2.PPH   3. Retained
                 4. Retained + PPH 5. Other

18 | |

INFANT   Sex; 1. Male   2. Female

19 | |

Apgar score (1 min)

20 21
| | |

Transferred to S.C.B.U.   1. Yes 2. No

22 | |

QUESTIONS TO MOTHER:

Was your husband/partner with you throughout labour and delivery? 1.Yes 2. No

23 | |

How soon after birth did you hold your baby?
            1. At once   2. Not at once but before leaving labour ward
            3. 1–4hours   4. 4–8 hours 5. More than 8 hours

24 | |

25 | |

Did you feed your baby in the labour ward?   1. Yes 2. No

26 | |

Did you plan this baby?   1. Yes 2. No

Your baby has been born in hospital, if possible would you have
preferred your baby to be born at home?
            1. Yes 2. No 3. Don't know

27 | |

Would your husband have preferred this baby to be born at home?
            1. Yes 2. No 3. Don't know

28 | |

Continued...........

LABOUR EXPERIENCE SCORES:

Experience of labour

Expectation score

Pain score

Feelings after delivery

Have any of the following events occurred during the last year?

A. Death of close family member   1.Yes 2. No

B. Changes in marriage situation 1.Yes 2. No

C. Illness/injury in close family 1.Yes 2. No

D. Changes in home situation   1. Yes 2. No

E. Changes in husbands employment 1.Yes 2. No

F. Other change mentioned by client

Who will look after you when you go home?

1. Husband   2. Husband+mother 3. Mother/in law
4. Friend/relative   5. No-one

Do you have close friends/relatives living nearby? 1. Yes 2. No

Did a midwife visit your home during ante-natal period? 1. Yes 2. No

Did you have a choice in length of stay in post-natal ward? 1. Yes 2. No

What kind of house do you live in?

1. Detached   2. Semi-detached 3. Terraced
4. Flat   5. Bed-sit   6. Other

Are you buying, renting or sharing with others as lodger?

1. Buying with mortgage   2. Renting
3. Sharing as lodger   4. Other

Any other comments

Likely date of transfer home/G.P.unit

130

Labour experience score sheets

I WOULD LIKE TO KNOW HOW YOU FEEL NOW ABOUT THE EXPERIENCE OF BIRTH

PLEASE TICK THE STATEMENT WHICH IS NEAREST TO HOW YOU FEEL

HAVING MY BABY WAS:

One of the worst experiences of my life	
Quite a bad experience	
An important experience, both good and bad	
Quite a good experience	
One of the best experiences of my life	

NOW THAT YOUR BABY IS BORN, DO YOU FEEL THAT THE EXPERIENCE OF LABOUR AND DELIVERY WAS:

Much better than I expected	
Better than I expected	
About as I expected it to be	
Worse than I expected	
Much worse than I expected	

THIS IS DIFFERENT, PLEASE MARK ON THIS "PAIN SCALE" WHERE YOU CONSIDER THAT YOUR EXPERIENCE OF PAIN IN LABOUR BELONGS:

Pain was unbearable most of the time   1   2   3   4   5   6   7   8   9   Pain never upset me during labour

HOW DID YOU FEEL IMMEDIATELY AFTER YOUR BABY WAS BORN?

Gloriously happy	
Tired but happy	
Relieved	
Too tired to care	
Disappointed	

Other comments

Unit No _____

Client No _____

Unit No. [1][2][3]

Client No [4][5][6]

Interview schedule (3) Hospital Midwife

Thinking of this mothers physical recovery from labour and delivery
do you consider that she;
        1. Recovered very well   2. Recovered quite well
        3. Did not recover as well as you would expect
        4. Still had not recovered at time of transfer

7 [ ]

Did she develop any physical problem after delivery? 1. Yes 2. No

8 [ ]

In YOUR opinion, what was this mothers emotional state during
her stay in the ward?   1. Very happy   2. Placid 3. Withdrawn
        4. Distressed   5. Mixture of moods 6. Other

9 [ ]

During her stay was she considered to have;
        1. "the baby blues"
        2. Distress due to known circumstances
        3. Abnormal emotional distress
        4. None of these

10 [ ]

Where distress was seen, at what stage of the post-natal perod was it seen?
.......................days

11 12 [ ][ ]

Comments;

How was the baby being fed at time of transfer?
        1. Breast only   2. Bottle only 3. Breast+ bottle

13 [ ]

Was there a change in feeding method during stay in ward?
        1. Yes 2. No 3. Don't know

14 [ ]

Did this mother get upset about the feeding? 1. Yes 2. No 3. Don't know

15 [ ]

How much help did this mother need with the feeding?
        1. A great deal of help 2. More than normal amount
        3. Normal amount of help 4. Less than normal amount
        5. Very little help needed

16 [ ]

How well did this mother manage her baby?
        1. Very well indeed 2. Quite well
        3. Did not manage very well
        4. Needed a great deal of help

17 [ ]

Did the baby develop any symptoms which needed medical attention?
        1. Yes 2. No

18 [ ]

Did the baby spend any time in S.C.B.U.
        1. Yes, before transfer to ward
        2. Yes, after initial transfer to ward
        3. All post-natal period spent in S.C.B.U.
        4. No

19 [ ]

Continued...........

Length of time infant spent in S.C.B.U. before transfer back to ward

      1. Less than 24 hours
      2. 24-48 hours
      3. More than 48 hours
      4. None

    20 ☐

During her stay in the ward, were any of the following seen?

      A. Tearfulness   1. Yes 2. No 3. Don't know
      B. Lack of sleep   1. Yes 2. No 3. Don't know
      C. Irritability   1. Yes 2. No 3. Don't know
      D. Undue fatigue   1. Yes 2. No 3. Don't know
      E. Poor appetite   1. Yes 2. No 3. Don't know

    21 22 ☐☐
    23 24 ☐☐
    25 ☐

What stage of the post-natal perod was this mother transferred?

      ....days

    26 27 ☐☐

To whose care was she transferred?

      1. Community midwife (Name & Tel No.........................⟩
      2. G.P.Unit (Name & Tel No...............................⟩
      3. Other

    28 ☐

Was this transfer arranged;

      1. By consultation before delivery
      2. After delivery
      3. Against medical/midwifery advice

    29 ☐

Observation of researcher;

    30 ☐

Were symptoms of distress noted in written/verbal reports? 1. Yes 2. No

Were symptoms reported during stay but not by interview midwife?

      1. Yes 2. No

    31 ☐

Did researcher notice distress which was not seen by staff?

      1. Yes 2. No

    32 ☐
    33 ☐

Did researcher notice distress which was ignored by staff? 1. Yes 2. No

Day of post-natal period distress was noted...............days

    34 35 ☐☐

Any other comments

    80 ☐ / 3

Questionnaire (1) Community Midwife

How soon after the mothers arrival home from hospital did she
receive the first visit from a midwife?

        1.During the same day on which she was transferred
        2.Morning after the day of transfer
        3.Afternoon of the day following transfer
        4.More than 24 hours after the day of transfer

                  7
               [ ]

Was this mother ever visited for more than once a day during the
post-natal period?
        1. Yes 2. No 3. Don't know

                  8
               [ ]

    if yes, please state if this was because of;
        1. Routine visiting pattern
        2. Mother needed extra attention
        3. Infant needed extra attention
        4. Other (please give details)
        ....

               9 10
           [ ][ ]
             11 12
           [ ][ ]

Did this mother show any of the following symptoms during the post-natal
period?

      1. Tearfulness 1. Yes 2. No 3. Don't know
      2. Lack of sleep 1. Yes 2. No 3. Don't know
      3. Irritability 1. Yes 2. No 3. Don't know
      4. Undue tiredness1. Yes 2. No 3. Don't know
      5. Poor appetite 1. Yes 2. No 3. Don't know

       13 14
     [ ][ ]
       15 16
     [ ][ ]
       17
     [ ]

In your opinion, how much support did this mother receive from her
family/ friends?
        1. Very good support
        2. Fairly good support
        3. Not enough support
        4. No support at all

            18
         [ ]

When you discharged this mother from the care of the midwifery
services, how was the baby being fed?
        1. Breast only
        2. Bottle only
        3. Combination of breast and bottle feeds

            19
         [ ]

Was there a change in feeding method after the mother came home
from hospital/G.P. unit? (Note; Do . not include change in make of baby milk)
        1. Yes 2. No

       20
     [ ]

How many different midwives attended this mother during the post-natal
period at home? (approximate number)

      ....

       21 22
     [ ][ ]

Did a health visitor also visit during the post-natal period?

        1. Yes 2. No 3. Don't know

       23
     [ ]

Continued...........

134

In your opinion, did this mother show signs of emotional distress
during the post-natal period at home?

24

> 1. Yes   2. No   3. Don't know

if yes, please give further details;

> A. In your opinion was this distress;
>
>> 1. "Baby blues"
>> 2. Distress due to particular circumstances
>> 3. Abnormal emotional distress
>> 4. None of these

25

> B. Were any of the factors listed below associated with
>   the distress?
>> 1. Family worries   1. Yes 2. No
>> 2. Physical discomfort   1. Yes 2. No
>> 3. Worried about the baby 1. Yes 2. No
>> 4. Other   1. Yes 2. No

26 27
28 29

> C. What stage of the post-natal period was distress seen?
>
> ....days

30 31

> D. Was this the day after her transfer home?
>
>> 1. Yes 2. No

32

How well do you think this mother was managing her baby when
you discharged from the care of the midwifery services?

> 1. Very well indeed
> 2. Quite well
> 3. Just managing to cope
> 4. Not managing at all well

33

Did you feel able to give this mother the kind of support you
felt that she needed?

> 1. Yes 2. No   3. Not sure

34

Please comment further if you wish

What stage of the post-natal period did you discharge this mother
from the care of the midwifery services?

> ....days

35 36

THANK YOU VERY MUCH FOR YOUR CO-OPERATION. IF THERE ARE ANY FURTHER
COMMENTS THAT YOU WISH TO ADD THESE WILL BE MOST WELCOME. PLEASE
WRITE THEM ON THE BACK OF THE QUESTIONNAIRE

PLEASE POST THIS QUESTIONNAIRE BACK TO ME IN THE STAMPED ADDRESSED
ENVELOPE AS SOON AS POSSIBLE.

80
5

Postnatal questionnaire (six weeks post delivery)
1) Hospital Care

Please put a tick in the square which is nearest to how <u>YOU</u> felt during your time in the ward. (Note: If you were transferred to another maternity unit/home please answer the statements as they apply to the unit you spent most time in)

Unit No.
Client No.

	STRONGLY AGREE	AGREE	NEITHER AGREE NOR DISAGREE	DISAGREE	STRONGLY DISAGREE	
1. I felt fit and well soon after my baby was born.						7
2. Feeding my baby was a worry.						8
3. I felt silly asking questions.						9
4. The midwives and nurses were helpful when I was feeding my baby.						10
5. I felt homesick and lonely.						11
6. The midwives and nurses seemed to understand what help I needed.						12
7. Different midwives gave different advice.						13
8. I didn't feel well enough to look after my baby.						14
9. Other mothers seemed to manage better than I did.						15
10. I needed more help in feeding my baby than I was given.						16
11. It was easy to get enough rest in the day-time.						17
12. Conflicting advice from midwives was upsetting.						18
13. I was helped to feel confident when feeding my baby.						19
14. I needed more rest at night.						20
15. It was easy to relax and feel at home.						21
16. Nobody listened to what I said, they just told me what to do.						22

Looking back on the time when your baby was born, do you think that the time you spent in hospital was:

Too long ☐   Too short ☐   About right ☐   23

Any further comments would be most welcome. Please use the back of this form.   80 6

2) *Community Care*

WHAT WAS IT LIKE FOR YOU WHEN YOU CAME HOME AND THE
DISTRICT MIDWIFE WAS CARING FOR YOU?

Unit No. | 1 | 2 | 3 |
         | 4 | 5 | 6 |

Client No.

. Please tick the square which is nearest to how YOU felt.

	STRONGLY AGREE	AGREE	NEITHER AGREE NOR DISAGREE	DISAGREE	STRONGLY DISAGREE	
1. Feeding the baby became easier, less of a worry.						7
2. After I came home, it was difficult to get enough rest.						8
3. The midwife seemed to understand what help I needed.						9
4. The family expected me to do too much.						10
5. I needed more help in feeding my baby than I was given.						11
6. Different midwives gave different advice.						12
7. I felt confident in handling my baby.						13
8. Too many people gave me advice.						14
9. The midwife always seemed to be in a hurry.						15
10. I felt I couldn't cope on my own.						16
11. My husband seemed to know what help I needed.						17
.. The Midwives visit was a great help.						18
13. The health visitor and the midwife gave conflicting advice.						19
14. There were too many different midwives visiting me.						20

If you have older children, please answer the next question:

	VERY WELL	QUITE WELL	DOESN'T MIND	NOT VERY WELL	BADLY	
How has your older child/children accepted the new baby?						21

Any further comments would be most welcome. Please use the back of this form.

80
7

Emotional well-being, satisfaction with motherhood and family support questionnaire

<u>THESE STATEMENTS ARE ABOUT HOW YOU FEEL NOW</u>

.There are no right or wrong answers to these statements.
Please tick the square which is nearest to how you feel now.

Unit No. | 1 | 2 | 3 |

Client No. | 4 | 5 | 6 |

	STRONGLY AGREE	AGREE	NEITHER AGREE NOR DISAGREE	DISAGREE	STRONGLY DISAGREE	
1. Most of the time, I feel happy and cheerful.						7
2. I feel confident about the way I cope.						8
3. I worry a lot.						9
4. Sometimes I feel I am a machine not a person.						10
5. I feel weepy at night.						11
6. I sleep well when the baby will let me.						12
7. I easily get upset if things go wrong.						13
8. The time I spend with my baby is the best part of the day.						14
9. I wish someone would tell me I'm doing a good job.						15
10. My family and friends are helpful.						16
11. I blame myself for problems with the baby.						17
12. I find it hard to make up my mind.						18
13. I talk to my baby quite a lot.						19
14. I don't enjoy food the way I used to.						20
15. I lose my temper more than I used to.						21
16. Sex doesn't interest me as much as before.						22
17. I feel full of energy these days.						23
18. I don't like to be left alone.						24
19. I've felt in low spirits since my baby was born.						25

Continued...........

	STRONGLY AGREE	AGREE	NEITHER AGREE nor DISAGREE	DISAGREE	STRONGLY DISAGREE	
20. Sometimes I feel as if the baby doesn't belong to me.						26
21. If I had more help I would manage better than I do.						27
22. I feel tired and weary.						28
23. I feel that my baby knows that I love him/her.						29
24. Sometimes I feel overwhelmed by all that I have to do.						30
25. Being a mother is satisfying.						31
26. Sometimes I wish I could go away on my own.						32
27. My husband gives me all the help I need him to give.						33
28. Getting my figure back is important to me.						34
29. If I need help, there is always someone I can turn to.						35
30. Caring for a small baby makes me feel nervous.						36
31. I enjoy stroking my baby's skin.						37
32. Sometimes I feel lonely and isolated.						38

Babies vary a great deal in the way they settle down to a routine. Now that your baby is a few weeks old, how do you feel that your baby compares with the average baby?

	BETTER THAN AVERAGE	ABOUT AVERAGE	WORSE THAN AVERAGE	
1. Number of crying spells.				39
2. Feeding difficulties.				
3. Sleeping pattern.				
4. Settling down to a predictable pattern of sleeping and feeding.				

Any further comments about how you feel now would be welcome. Please use the back of the form.

THANK YOU SO MUCH FOR YOUR HELP IN THIS PROJECT. I DO HOPE THAT YOU HAVE ENJOYED TAKING PART. PLEASE POST THE QUESTIONNAIRE BACK TO ME AS SOON AS POSSIBLE.

80

8